THE
BRIDE'S
GUIDE TO GLOW

THE
BRIDE'S
GUIDE TO GLOW

EVERYTHING YOU NEED
for BEAUTIFUL SKIN
on YOUR BIG DAY

TARREN BROOKS

CHRONICLE BOOKS
SAN FRANCISCO

Library of Congress Cataloging-in-Publication Data available.

ISBN 978-1-4521-8337-4

Manufactured in China.

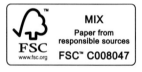

Design by AJ Hansen.
Typeset in Columbia Sans, Mrs Eaves, and Brandon Grotesque.

10 9 8 7 6 5 4 3 2 1

Chronicle books and gifts are available at special quantity
discounts to corporations, professional associations, literacy
programs, and other organizations. For details and discount
information, please contact our premiums department at
corporatesales@chroniclebooks.com or at 1-800-759-0190.

Chronicle Books LLC
680 Second Street
San Francisco, California 94107
www.chroniclebooks.com

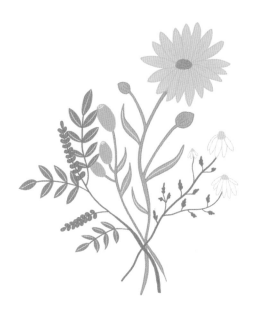

"Holistic skin care is cultivating a mindful pattern of self-care to improve skin health and well-being"
—Katie Woods

CONTENTS

INTRODUCTION

You and your skin have been on a long journey together. Since birth, your skin has been a virtual mirror of the inner workings of your body, signaling to you what is going on internally. And it's the first part of you that people see, the way you greet and are presented to the world.

My skin and I have been on our own unique journey, involving a career of fussing around with varied techniques and products. What feels like a lifetime ago, I worked at a makeup counter selling pore-clogging foundation and terrible perfumes. At the time, that was considered high-end beauty, but the cosmetics were filled with terrible ingredients. I was unknowingly depositing nasty compounds into my body, and encouraging customers to do the same. These products wreaked havoc on my skin.

I didn't understand the trouble I was causing until I changed career paths and my skin started detoxing all the harmful ingredients I had been using. Applying all those silicones, parabens, and phthalates resulted in acne I had never had before, plus scarring and hyperpigmentation issues. These problems took a while to sort out. During that time, I learned how to care for my skin topically with simple, clean products, nourish my skin with my diet, and combat skin issues in the healthiest ways.

This discovery sparked my interest in holistic skin care and led me to pursue a profession in the field. After becoming a licensed esthetician, I dove deep into holistic esthetics. I took courses in formulating organic skin-care products, learned specific treatment techniques, and studied herbalism and nutrition. Now, through my work, I strive every day to help people detoxify their skin-care routines. I have helped brides achieve clear skin after struggling with everything from acne to hyperpigmentation. I find deep joy in helping people feel and look their best for big events, and for daily life. There is nothing that makes me happier than receiving a message from a client letting me know they are feeling confident in their skin and have completely given up makeup, or their skin is looking the best it ever has.

I am here to help you **GLOW**. I am passionate about skin care, in part because I know firsthand the problems that cheap, toxic products can create. This book offers a holistic approach to skin care by showing you how to nourish your face, mind, and body before the wedding. By taking into account your whole body, you can identify what is going on with different systems and how that shows through in your skin. Oftentimes, if there is a skin disorder, it means there is an underlying issue at hand. Unmanaged stress, poor nutrition, and lack of sleep all have a negative impact on the function of our bodies, and the skin can sometimes be the first indicator when a system in the body needs extra attention. Soothing and healing from the inside out is necessary for our best skin, so I offer ways in which you can support your skin's natural functions and nourish it from the inside. You'll also find several routines to promote glowing skin in the lead-up to your wedding, as well as tips for dealing with skin-related emergencies on the big day.

There is a lot of pressure to look "perfect" for your "perfect wedding," to solidify your "perfect relationship." If you are thinking that everything must be perfect, please let go of that notion and the pressure that comes with it. (And if you're not thinking that, great. You're already one step ahead!) The truth is, the stress of perfection will cause just that . . . stress. Unnecessary, harmful stress. Part of glowing skin, as you will learn, is stress management.

MANAGED STRESS = MENTAL HEALTH = GLOW

Remember, your partner wants to marry **YOU**, not some cosmetically altered, stressed-out version of you. We are imperfect beings, and you will be doing yourself and your skin a huge favor if you embrace that! It is important to accept the skin you have and focus on healing, enhancing, and supporting it. Not fixing it. Your skin is an extension of you. Learn to love it.

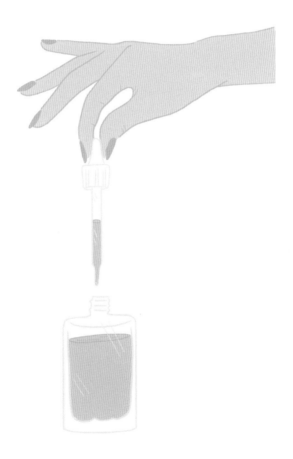

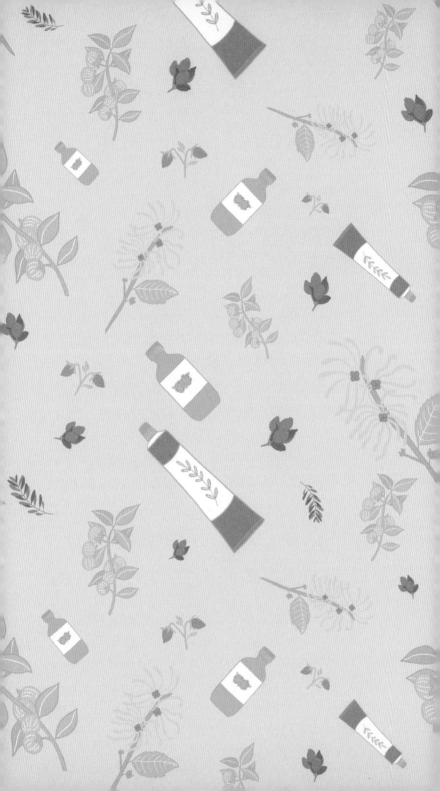

SKIN CARE
AND
ROUTINES

Our skin is our largest organ and very in tune with the rest of our body. Caring for your skin daily with the proper routines is mandatory for glow. It takes time and focus to determine what your skin is telling you it needs. Although you are shedding millions of cells a day, your skin is with you for life. I talk a lot about the skin on the face, but do not forget skin is full body! All of it needs your attention and has differing needs.

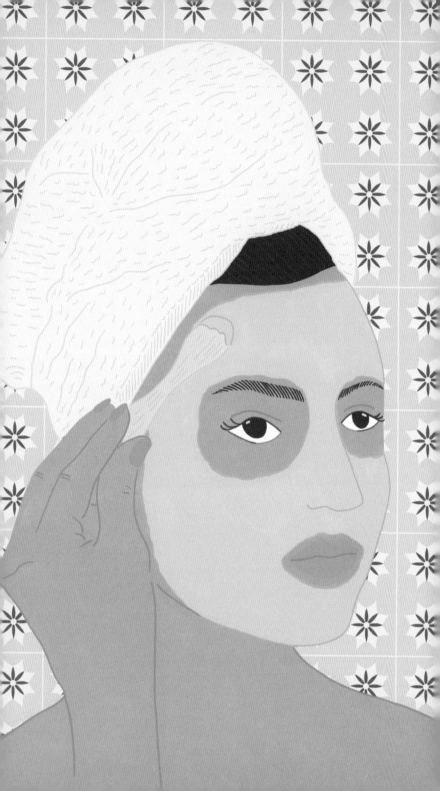

Skin Characteristics

Think of your skin as having characteristics (often called conditions). What do you like about your skin and wish to highlight? What do you wish to balance? The basis of a healthy skin-care routine is discovering the right products to work with your skin's natural functions and unique qualities.

Your skin characteristics are determined by your individual genetic makeup and ethnic background. Skin also changes periodically, depending on the time of year, weather, your menstrual cycle, geographical location, products, stress levels, and so on. The notion of having "dry," "combo," or "oily" skin and falling in line with everyone else who shares this type is an idea of the past. Our skin is much more nuanced than labels suggest. These generic skin-type terms are mostly used for marketing purposes, which can be helpful at times, but are vastly oversimplified. Skin can possess some of these qualities, like "dry" or "oily," but that does not truly define how it should be treated. Although your composition generally remains the same, skin should be treated according to different characteristics, like the ones highlighted here.

If your skin is **SENSITIVE**, there is a presence of redness and reactivity. Redness will often increase with friction or heat. Broken capillaries may be present. Physical exfoliation, like scrubs, should not be used; apply only chemical exfoliants like enzymes and acids. These exfoliants should be used with caution and in small amounts at first. Cleansing should be done lightly, possibly using just water or an oil cleanser instead of a deeper cleanser that works to saponify oils. Saponifying is the act of turning excess oil into soap. Use simple, nonaggressive products throughout your routine. Focus on soothing the skin, and watch out for internal triggers such as stress, diet, or sluggish digestion.

DRY skin will look more textured and tight, have slow elastic recoil, and even be flaky. Fine lines or wrinkles are more apparent when skin is lacking hydration and/or moisture. Internal hydration is key, so be sure you are drinking enough water. Externally, there should be an emphasis on introducing both hydration (water) and moisture (oil) to the skin, via products. These can look like moisturizing creams, or better yet, a hydrosol and then a replenishing oil blend. Oils used for dry skin can be heavier or have a larger molecular structure. Dry skin should always be treated gently because the ability to collect and distribute nourishment may be compromised. The goal with dry skin is not only to hydrate by drinking water, but to build and maintain the skin's own ability to moisturize.

If your skin is often **OILY**, that likely means there is an excess of sebum on the skin that needs to be reduced. This will look like extra shine and clogged pores, and if you wiped your face, oil would come off. Many times, products for oily skin will destroy the skin's microbiome, leaving the skin feeling "squeaky clean" but robbing the skin of its acid mantle. The acid mantle is a layer of sebum and sweat—an essential protective barrier. Stay away from "oil-free" products or over-stripping cleansers, which focus on withdrawing the oils from your skin, as these can backfire and cause an overproduction of sebum. If skin is oily all over, alpha hydroxy acids and beta hydroxy acids can be used in small amounts. The skin should be treated with balancing oils like jojoba, sunflower, and safflower. The objective with oily skin is to decrease the production of oil but leave enough of it to maintain healthy moisture and function.

A lot of people think they have acne, when their skin only has occasional breakouts. If your skin is truly **ACNEIC**, blemishes are always present and skin is generally inflamed. Oftentimes this includes large whiteheads and cystic, painful lesions. Skin should be treated gently and hormones should be checked. The wrong product regimen, internal inflammation, hormonal imbalances, and dietary sensitivities can all exacerbate acneic skin. Too much bacteria can lead to acne, so a healthy routine is essential. With acneic skin, find triggers and minimize them, whether they are internal or external. Also keep down general inflammation in the body, which might mean avoiding certain foods, excessive heat, and stress.

For skin that feels **FLAKY AND DULL** and is not sensitive, a good exfoliation is in order. A physical exfoliant like a washcloth, facial dry brush, gentle scrub, or microderm-abrasion treatment could help slough off dry, dead surface skin cells. If your skin is flaking and sensitive, be very gentle and avoid physical exfoliation beyond light pressure with a soft washcloth. Flaky, dull skin should be exfoliated regularly to ensure cellular turnover.

HYPERPIGMENTED, or sun-damaged skin, is characterized by discoloration. Sun protection is of the utmost importance to help maintain an even tone and keep from activating excess melanin. Antioxidants are crucial for repairing cells and fighting free radicals. With time, powerful antioxidants can both prevent and reverse hyperpigmentation, resulting in more even skin tone.

BLEMISHED skin will have an occasional breakout, but that does not always equal acne. I often see clients with breakouts around the chin area or jawline. These typically occur right before or during menstruation, due to hormonal changes. Foods in your diet can also be a cause, with three main triggers: dairy, gluten, and sugar. These breakouts tend to happen on the cheeks or forehead. Blemished skin should never be picked at. It should be treated with spot treatments, and physical exfoliants should be avoided when breakouts are present. The intention here is to keep blemishes healing swiftly and prevent them from coming back. Much like with acneic skin, minimizing triggers is essential.

When treating skin that shares both dry and oily areas, often referred to as **COMBINATION** skin, balance is key. Combination skin produces excess oil in the T-zone (chin, nose, and forehead) and dryness in the cheeks. Be sure neither area is being starved of what it needs. Balancing products work best, such as gentle cleansers and light oils. You can use different products in different areas of the face, but this is unnecessary and extra work. Avoid excessive cleansing or exfoliation.

Your skin most likely has overlapping traits, and taking care of your skin is all about finding the harmony within those traits. If you are confused about your skin characteristics, an esthetician can help determine what will work best for you in the allotted time before your wedding.

DETERMINE YOUR
SKIN CONDITION

*Keep in mind that your skin probably
possesses multiple characteristics.*

Does your skin feel dry when
you wake up in the morning?
IF YES, **YOUR SKIN IS DEHYDRATED**

Does your skin feel dry throughout the day?
IF YES, **YOUR SKIN IS DRY**

Does your skin have a lot of freckles or areas that
are darker than the rest of your face? Do these
areas get slightly darker with heat and/or sun?
IF YES, **YOUR SKIN IS HYPERPIGMENTED**

Does your skin have some oily areas
and some dry?
IF YES, **YOUR SKIN IS COMBINATION**

Is your skin reactive, or does it
have a tendency to get red?
IF YES, **YOUR SKIN MAY BE SENSITIVE**

Does your skin look oily throughout
the day or in the afternoon?
IF YES, **YOUR SKIN IS OILY**

Do you get occasional breakouts?
IF YES, **YOUR SKIN IS BLEMISHED**

Do you have constant breakouts?
IF YES, **YOUR SKIN IS ACNEIC**

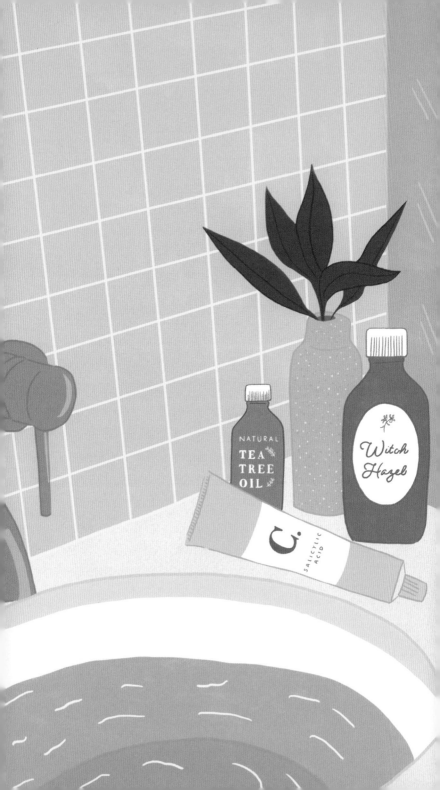

Pimples

Pimples happen when a sebaceous (oil) gland is blocked and infected. This infection leads to a swollen, red lesion filled with pus. This process is your skin's natural defense system to protect itself and treat infection. Our hormones activate our sebaceous glands, which is why we have blemishes pop up when we are in puberty, stressed, or menstruating. Dietary and environmental triggers can also play a role in sebaceous activity. Pimples are best cared for with a localized spot treatment and left alone until they are gone. It is best to soothe and aid in healing, and resist the urge to interfere beyond this.

To soothe, keep the affected area cool and avoid using heavy oils or scrubbing. If the area is red and swollen, indirect cold, such as an ice cube wrapped with a towel, can ease the swelling. Salicylic acid is a beneficial chemical exfoliant since it is anti-inflammatory and will activate cellular renewal. Tea tree oil is a popular remedy but should always be diluted with a solution like witch hazel. Essential oils, like tea tree, are the strongest plant extracts available, and most are too active to be put directly onto the skin. Tea tree oil is antibacterial and antimicrobial, but it can also be very drying and possibly cause more of a breakout. As a rule of thumb, use two parts witch hazel to one part tea tree oil.

Avoid picking or popping pimples and blackheads. When squeezed, these lesions can burst, which may release pressure but also causes a trauma to the skin. We have all done it. It can be tough to wake up with a huge zit staring back at you from the mirror, but they are best left alone. There really is no good reason to pick. Would you rather have a scab for a week or two and possibly a long-lasting scar or a pimple that will fade after a day or two? Compulsive picking is often a symptom of anxiety, and the energy should be directed elsewhere.

Rupturing a lesion may be the number one cause of pimples. Have you ever discovered a blemish, "popped" the blemish, and the next day woken up with a new blemish nearby? That's because you have spread bacteria, if not on top of the skin, *in* the dermis. You may have disturbed an infection, and it has spread to a nearby pore. One to two monthly hormonal spots can easily turn into a month-long breakout by constant picking. Picking also increases your chances of scarring, or at best, makes the blemish take much longer to heal. The best way to treat a blemish is with a well-balanced spot treatment, left on overnight. Ideally a spot treatment is anti-inflammatory and lightly exfoliating. Contact a skin-care professional if you have a whitehead that lasts longer than a week.

Two percent of the population suffers from excoriation disorder, or dermatillomania, a compulsive picking disorder that interrupts healthy skin and daily life. This disorder is typically related to obsessive compulsive disorder and/or social anxiety. If this sounds like you, please seek professional help, preferably from a psychologist and an esthetician.

Tips for avoiding blemished skin:

+ Keep skin clean with the appropriate cleanser for your skin, since bacteria buildup can lead to pimples. Refer to page 26 for help finding the right type of cleanser.

+ Regularly exfoliate to keep debris and excess sebum from building up in the pores. See page 40 for information on exfoliators.

+ Identify and eliminate dietary triggers altogether, or keep them to a minimum. This will take a little work involving tuning in to your body and how it reacts to different foods. Go to page 72 for more information on dietary triggers.

+ Clean makeup brushes after every use; they can be a breeding ground for bacteria. I lather the brushes with a drop of baby shampoo and water, rinse well, and then leave them flat to dry.

+ Wash pillowcases once a week. I suggest using silk pillowcases, as they are hypoallergenic and can be more breathable.

Facial Skin-Care Habits

Skin thrives with proper nourishment, topically and internally, and routine is essential for maintaining a healthy complexion. Pre-wedding, a routine will instill balance during a time when a schedule is interrupted with factors such as travel or stress. Then, when the big day arrives, you will already have systems in place for looking your best. Routine not only promotes clear skin but internal well-being—a welcome respite during a stressful time. You cannot wash your face once a week and expect glowing skin. Creating a skin-care routine to support specific skin needs—and sticking to it—is important. Choosing the right products is foundational when establishing a routine. When you shop for skin-care products or see a professional, feel free to request samples, but keep in mind that it can take a month or even two to really see results. If your skin reacts poorly, consult your esthetician. It may be an issue your skin is working out, or it could be an indication of a bigger problem, such as a reaction to a product. (It's rare, but it can happen!)

Take the time to establish a routine that you love. Invest in fewer, better products that resonate with you and work for your skin. Create a ritual around it. Use it as your time to get away from all the planning and stressing. Take a full minute to really massage the cleanser into your skin, 5 minutes to do an at-home steam, or 20 to enjoy a face mask. Check in with yourself, and tune in to your body.

Basic Skin-Care Routine

An ideal routine consists of cleansing, toning, moisturizing, and applying an eye treatment and sun protection. Supplemental skin care can include serums, masks, or exfoliators. This section outlines a basic, ideal routine you can put in place now and continue long after your wedding is over. The following section expands on supplemental treatments you might want to add to your routine before your wedding for maximum glow.

A few quick notes before we get started:

- Skin can require different remedies based on where you live or what season it is. For example, if you live in a dry region or at high altitude, you may need to double up on your moisturizer and carry a lip balm with you at all times; on the other hand, during a humid summer, you may need to use a more astringent cleanser to remove excess sebum.

- You should only introduce ingredients that you can pronounce and recognize — preferably plant based and whole plant.

- You should perform your routine in the morning and again at night, possibly switching up products for different times of the day.

- Treat your neck and décolletage the same way you treat your face. The skin in those areas is fragile and can show damage quickly, so it deserves just as much attention!

CLEANSERS

The first step of a skin-care routine is cleansing. Your skin collects makeup, dirt, sebum, dead skin cells, and general pollutants throughout the day. Cleansing removes all this debris and balances out the pH of your skin. Soaps and cleansers saponify your excess oil on the skin. A good cleanser is gentle on the skin and doesn't strip you of your own moisture but is still very effective. If your esthetician thinks adding an exfoliating acid to your skin-care routine is a good idea, a cleanser is a great way to do that. Exfoliating acids are used to loosen the bond between cells in the epidermis. These can be small or large percentages of acids. It is always ideal to sample first, before buying.

Some cleansers require you to wet your face beforehand; others are applied to dry skin. Take time to massage the cleanser into your skin. Massage gently, focusing on areas that are more oily or have blemishes. Make sure you get your hairline and jawline. Take a full minute to do this. Time yourself, if that's helpful. Cleansers should leave your skin feeling soft and refreshed. If a cleanser leaves you feeling "squeaky clean," or dry and tight, this is an indication that it's not the right cleanser for you. Cleansers that yield these results are stripping you of your skin's natural oils and will do more damage than good.

There are several types of cleansing methods:

OIL CLEANSING is using an oil-based cleanser or a pure oil to cleanse. Jojoba oil or grapeseed oil are great for this, and you can find them wherever skin-care oils are sold. There are also more targeted blends of oils, labeled oil cleansers. Cleansing with oil can be very helpful for balancing the skin's oil production and keeping pores clean. It can be done daily, or a few times per week. Whatever works best for your skin, just be sure to keep it consistent. Oil cleansing works for all skin types, balancing oil in both dry and oily skin.

BALM CLEANSING is similar to oil cleansing, just using a balm specially formulated to cleanse.

CREAM CLEANSERS are typically used for drier skin. This cleanser is massaged into the skin and then rinsed with water. Cream cleansers are beneficial for more sensitive or compromised skin, as they minimally influence the balance of oils and can be very calming and nourishing to the skin.

GEL AND FOAMING CLEANSERS work to remove impurities. Gels are thick and have a jelly-like consistency. They are great for more sensitive, acne-prone skin because they will saponify oils but not be as stripping as a foaming cleanser. Foaming cleansers that are not for-mulated with foaming agents (sulfates) can be helpful when a deeper cleanse is needed. However, these should be alternated with a more gentle cleanser.

MICELLAR WATER is a cleansing water that is lightweight and unique because it is not rinsed or wiped away. It stays on the surface of the epidermis, which can be problematic for skin prone to acne or breakouts. These formulas are made up of surfactant molecules suspended in balls of water called micelles. They are used with a cotton ball or pad. I would not suggest micellar water as a daily cleanser. It is best suited when you need to clean your face in a pinch, like when you need to remove makeup before a workout but don't want to do a third cleanse of the day. Because of the heavy water content, these cleansers require quite a bit of preservatives, so if you choose this cleansing route, make sure the preservatives used are nontoxic.

MECHANICAL CLEANSING BRUSHES are something I would avoid using. I have seen them destroy capillaries, prematurely age skin, fuel breakouts, and cause loss of pigmentation. These problems typically start in the cheeks, where the skin is the thinnest and most vulnerable. If you are using mechanical brushes, transition to a soft, manual brush and keep it gentle.

TONERS

A **TONER** should always be used immediately after cleansing and before any serums or moisturizers. A toner's traditional job is to balance the pH of the skin; pH stands for "potential of hydrogen," in other words, the acidity or alkalinity. This is measured on a scale of 1 to 14, 1 being the most acidic, 7 being neutral, and 14 being the most alkaline. The skin's pH hovers around 5.5, which is slightly acidic. A toner's goal is to bring the pH of the skin to the healthy state of 5.5. Toners have evolved and can now be formulated to introduce other active ingredients to aid the skin. Toners can be filled with hydrating ingredients or exfoliants, or they can be really simple and made mostly of witch hazel or hydrosols. These are all great! Toners are unsung heroes in the skin-care world. Even a simple toning solution, with one to three ingredients, can make a huge difference in the skin's tone and texture.

HYDROSOLS, such as rose water, have toning qualities and can be used as toners. They are also known as hydrolats. Hydrosols are the distillation by-product of essential oils. They are pure distilled water, leaving some residual microscopic essential oils suspended in the water. Used on their own, or blended into other formulas, hydrosols bring a light, fleeting scent and have been known to enhance a person's mood. Hydrosols are great when more active ingredients are not necessary or are irritating. I love the simplicity of hydrosols and the water content they bring, which is especially important when using an oil as a moisturizer since the oil carries no water, as a cream or lotion would. Moisturization of the skin depends on the balance between oil and water, and a hydrosol is a great way to add water to your skin. Skin thrives with simplicity. When you work with the skin and simply support its own systems, which are already in place, your skin will thrive.

MOISTURIZERS

Our skin has a way of balancing its own water and lipids. Everyone's skin has a delicate balance of moisture (oil) and hydration (water). Our bodies are so brilliant, constantly coordinating all systems to achieve balance and the best health possible, but they still require our support. Adding extra moisture reduces the chances of skin issues with both dry and oily skin. A moisturizer also protects our skin from the elements.

A moisturizer helps maintain a healthy amount of oil and water. Moisturizers can be creams, lotions, balms, or oils. **CREAMS AND LOTIONS** are moisturizers formulated with a blend of oil and water. In order for these two ingredients to be blended together, there must be an emulsifying agent present. Unfortunately, creams and lotions are not always beneficial for the skin. Water is a breeding ground for bacteria. So when a water element is present, there must be preservatives in the formulation. If you wish to use a cream or lotion, stick to a product with fewer ingredients in the list. Unnecessary ingredients, typically only added to enhance the look and feel of the product, can worsen skin conditions.

There is a range of **OILS**; some are best for oily skin and some are best for dry skin. Which oil will work for you depends on the weight of the different oils. If you are going out on your own, I recommend a pure, organic jojoba oil as a good place to start. Jojoba oil mimics our skin's own lipids and promotes homeostasis, or stability within the tissues of the skin. If you find jojoba oil feels too heavy and leaves an oily-feeling residue on the face, try something with a lighter weight. Grapeseed or rose hip are great options. If jojoba oil leaves you feeling dry, try something with more weight to keep you dewy throughout the day, like hemp or almond oil. And always use a hydrosol or water-heavy toner underneath an oil so that your skin is getting water-based moisture as well.

BALMS that are used as skin moisturizers are a blend of oil thickened into a solid with a wax. Balms operate much like an oil, delivering lipids and maintaining balance. The added wax helps to seal in moisture, while still letting the skin breathe. These types of moisturizers are particularly protective and healing.

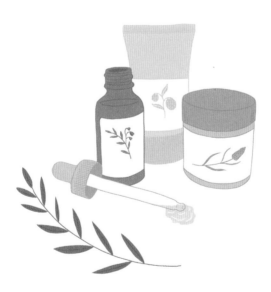

	OIL	TO TREAT
	Almond, sweet (*Prunus amygdalus dulcis*)	Dry, sensitive, irritated, red, itchy skin
	Apricot kernel (*Prunus armeniaca*)	Dry, sensitive skin, fine lines and wrinkles, sagging; good for skin with dryness and oiliness
	Rose hip (*Rosa moschata*)	Oily or dry skin, wrinkles, fine lines, hyperpigmentation, acne, scarring
	Grapeseed (*Vitis vinifera*)	Acne-prone and oily skin
	Jojoba (*Simmondsia chinensis*)	All skin conditions, particularly combination, perioral dermatitis, eczema, and psoriasis
	Hemp seed (*Cannabis sativa*)	Inflamed, dry, or damaged skin

BENEFITS

Good source of vitamin E, vitamin K, omega-3s, and omega-6s. Soothing and moisturizing, while still having a light feel.

Good source of vitamin E, omega-3s, and omega-6s. Helps improve elasticity with a tightening effect. Absorbs quickly.

High vitamin A and vitamin C content. Regenerative. Promotes collagen formation. Can reduce scar tissue and UV damage.

Contains vitamin E and omega-6s. Lightweight and absorbs easily into skin. Full of antioxidants. Tightening and toning.

Technically a fatty ester, this liquid wax can be used as an oil for its anti-inflammatory, balancing, and nourishing traits.

Balancing, anti-inflammatory, and antioxidant rich.

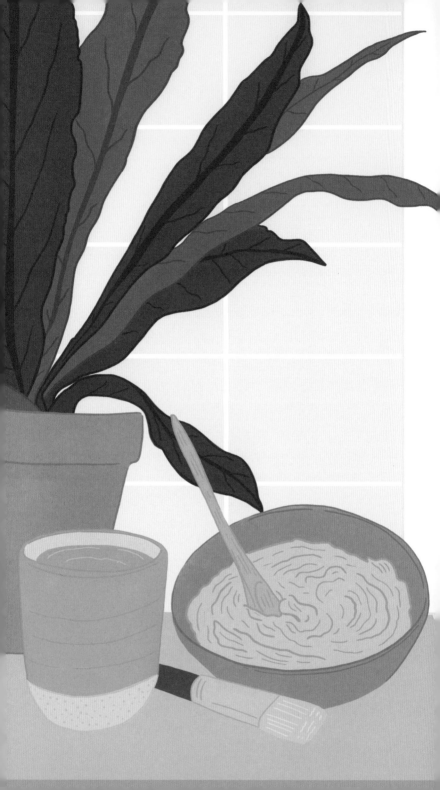

Additional Skin-Care Steps

EYE TREATMENTS

The skin around the eyes is very delicate and requires extra attention. Skin-care brands formulate products for this specific area and type of skin. These products are lighter and may contain targeted ingredients to treat fine lines, wrinkles, puffiness, or dark circles. In an eye-care product, caffeine, like coffee bean extract or green tea, stimulates blood and lymph flow and can help cells metabolize fat, reducing enlarged bags under the eyes and dark circles. Peptides or vitamin A can combat fine lines and wrinkles. Eye creams should be applied in very small amounts, and only on the boned ridge of the eye area, not on the eyelid or too close to the eye.

Green tea bags are great for de-puffing and "waking up" the eye area. To do this, steep two tea bags, remove them from the water, and wait until they're cool in temperature. Squeeze out the excess water and apply one to each eye for 5 minutes.

If you drink too much at your rehearsal dinner or bachelorette party, brighten your eyes with homeopathic eye drops, ideally containing the herb eyebright (*Euphrasia officinalis*). Puffiness can be reduced by moving lymph with an at-home massage.

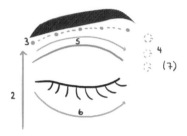

Here is an at-home massage routine to remedy puffiness or dark circles:

1. After cleansing, toning, and moisturizing, use the eye treatment product of your choice. Use twice as much eye product as you normally would (still a small amount).

2. With the pads of your two forefingers, move straight upward along your nose until you hit your brow bone, just under where your eyebrow starts.

3. Apply light to medium pressure here and hold for 5 seconds. Do the same thing, 5 times, working outward under the eyebrow. Be gentle with the skin in this area; you do not need to be forceful to move lymph.

4. Create light circular motions on the temple, using slightly more pressure on the downstroke of the

circle. Repeat this motion in front of the ears, moving down just under the jawbone and then continuing down the neck to the collarbone.

5. Then, again with the pads of your forefingers, use light pressure to create a sweeping motion just under the eyebrow. Do this 5 times.

6. Use light pressure to create a sweeping motion under the eye, under where the puffiness is. Do this 5 times.

7. Repeat step 4.

SIMPLE LIP SCRUB

1 pea-size dollop   1 pinch sugar
lip balm

1. Take a dollop of lip balm and a pinch of sugar. Mix together.
2. Scrub for 1 minute and rinse.

This can be done once a week and even the night before your wedding. Follow with a balm and pucker up!

LIP TREATMENTS

Do not forget your lips! The skin on our lips is extra sensitive and has the proclivity to become dry and even cracked. Treat your lips kindly with a lip balm, hopefully one with an SPF that will protect your lips from the sun. A good lip balm contains natural oils and a wax, like beeswax. Shea butter is usually too heavy for the face, but perfect for the lips. Apply as needed. Lips can become reliant on the moisture of a lip balm, so if you feel as if your lips are no longer benefitting, it may be time to take a break. If your lips are dry, create a simple lip scrub.

SERUMS

Serums are targeted treatment products used in addition to a basic skin-care routine. Serums are built to address very specific skin-care concerns, such as softening fine lines, combatting sun damage, increasing hydration, soothing acne, or toning down redness. They are packed with active ingredients to suit your needs and are typically designed to penetrate deeper into the epidermis than a moisturizer. Serums are worn throughout the day and should be layered on after your toner and before your moisturizer.

MASKS

Masks are made to enhance skin. Much like serums, they are targeted for specific skin concerns and conditions. Usually they are applied onto clean skin and then removed 10 to 20 minutes later. Masks have different bases, such

AT-HOME FACE MASKS

HYDRATING MASK FOR DRY SKIN

1 Tbsp honey

¼ Tbsp olive oil

¼ Tbsp colloidal oatmeal

SOOTHING MASK FOR INFLAMED SKIN

¼ avocado, mashed

1 Tbsp honey

¼ tsp ground chamomile

CLARIFYING MASK FOR ACNEIC OR BLEMISHED SKIN

½ Tbsp cosmetic grade white clay (found at your local health food store or online at mountainroseherbs .com)

½ Tbsp hydrosol, honey, or fruit puree (melons, strawberries, blueberries)

¼ tsp spirulina

1. Mix the ingredients for your desired mask until they reach a spreadable consistency, adding more olive oil, honey, or fruit puree, as needed. Then spread the mixture onto your face.

2. Leave the mask on for 5 to 20 minutes, making sure it does not dry.

3. Rinse your face with warm water, pat dry, and follow with a toner and moisturizer.

as clay, hyaluronic acid, and honey. A mask should never dry on your skin. If you can feel it drying, splash your face with water to keep it damp, or take it off altogether. When a mask dries, it may be drawing water from your skin, leaving your skin dry and dehydrated.

Sheet masks have become very popular and can be found almost anywhere. A face-shaped piece of fabric, soaked in a blend of active ingredients, is applied and left on for a short period of time. The occlusive nature of the mask ensures the active ingredients are trapped against your skin. This method is particularly useful as a hydrating mask, but be careful that the ingredients in the mask are ones you would like pressed to your skin for 20 minutes. I am a fan of hyaluronic acid–based masks. Hyaluronic acid is a hydrating acid (rather than an exfoliating acid like an AHA or BHA). Hyaluronic acid works to bind water to the skin, delivering quick, short-term hydration.

EXFOLIATORS

Exfoliating—sloughing off dry, dead surface skin cells, or excess oil—is important for skin health. Removing residue hidden in the pores is crucial to keeping skin radiant. Our skin cells turn over or renew themselves in a process called desquamation. This process takes about 28 days, slowing down as we age. Exfoliation treatments speed the rate at which cells turn over and encourage new, healthy skin cells. Skin conditions will determine the best method of exfoliation.

Frequency of exfoliation depends on how much your skin can handle, and the type of exfoliation you use. The most common issue I see in my practice is the overuse of exfoliation products. Well-meaning brides-to-be are scrubbing their skin raw and creating new problems.

BOTANICAL EXFOLIANT

1 Tbsp cosmetic grade white clay (found at your local health food store or online at mountainroseherbs .com)

¼ Tbsp finely ground oats

¼ Tbsp poppy seeds

1. Mix the ingredients together and slowly trickle in water or a hydrosol; blend until a watery paste is created.

2. Massage into clean skin for 30 seconds and rinse with warm water.

3. Pat dry with a clean towel before toning and moisturizing.

This is a great physical exfoliant, but if your skin is sensitive, you may want to seek out something else.

Over-exfoliation can spread bacteria, causing acne, or even worse, it can thin the skin and create sensitivity or premature aging. A rule of thumb is to be gentle—less is more.

There are two different types of exfoliants—chemical and physical. Chemical exfoliation involves enzymes and alpha-hydroxy acids or beta-hydroxy acids, often referred to as AHAs or BHAs. These exfoliants create a chemical reaction to loosen the bond between cells in the epidermis. Chemical exfoliants can be found in masks, serums, cleansers, and toners. Exfoliants in cleansers and masks may have a higher concentration, as they are on the skin for a short period of time before removal. When exfoliants are in a serum or toner, they are a lower percentage but stay on the skin longer, slowly and gently working to turn cells over.

Physical exfoliants are scrubs or tools with a texture for physically removing dead surface skin cells. These types of exfoliants are rough in texture and are not meant for people with broken capillaries, an active breakout, or any sort of skin sensitivity. The rough texture can aggravate these skin conditions.

The kind of exfoliant you use depends entirely on your skin and its current state. Physical exfoliants are a good option if your skin is clear. They can be used occasionally if you feel a rough texture that needs to be removed, or if you have skin that is dry and flaky, but not inflamed. A facial sponge or almond scrub is a great option for gently exfoliating dry skin. The downside, as mentioned earlier, is they can dig into the skin and cause irritation. Chemical exfoliants can also be irritating, but when used in the right percentages and amounts for your skin type, they can be used more frequently (sometimes daily!). They are ideal for people with inflammation, acne, dryness, fine lines and wrinkles, and oiliness. Salicylic acid is a good general purpose chemical exfoliant since it has an anti-inflammatory effect. Glycolic acid is another good option, especially for acneic skin. Just be sure to use it gently. Do not exfoliate over broken skin; doing so can delay healing. When using any new exfoliant, start slow and ensure you are protected from the sun afterward.

It is important to exfoliate regularly and also before an event. Exfoliating will make sure your skin is as clear and bright as possible. If you plan to use an exfoliant before your wedding, make sure to try it out when you do not have something coming up, and again before your engagement party, bachelorette, and bridal shower—*so you know how your skin will react!*

FACIAL STEAMING

Take a few minutes to relax and simultaneously improve your skin with a botanical facial steam. Steam opens up the pores and gives a deep cleanse. Inhaling steam can also clear congestion in the sinuses and lungs, and calm the nervous system. By adding dried herbs to the steam, you not only create a lovely aromatherapy experience but also add even more great benefits for your skin.

SELF-LOVE HERBAL STEAM

¼ cup [20 g] licorice root (*Glycyrrhiza glabra*)

¼ cup [15 g] calendula (*Calendula officinalis*)

¼ cup [10 g] chamomile (*Matricaria chamomilla*)

¼ cup [15 g] rose hip (*Rosa canina*)

---

1. Bring 2 to 3 quarts [1.8 to 2.8 L] of water to a boil. Add the herbs. Simmer for 5 minutes while you go wash your face. (Wait to tone and moisturize until after steaming.)

2. Remove the pot from the heat.

3. Drop a towel over your head and the pot, keeping your face at least 10 inches [25 cm] away from the water at all times. *If you are any closer, you can burn your skin.*

4. Close your eyes, take some deep breaths, and relax.

5. Steam for no longer than 7 minutes!

6. When finished, rinse your face with warm water.

Variation: Add or remove herbs depending on your skin's needs. You want about 1 cup [60 g] total of dried herbs.

HERBS TO USE		BENEFITS
	Marshmallow root (*Althaea officinalis*) Elderflower (*Sambucus*) Rose hip (*Rosa canina*)	Hydrating
	Sage (*Salvia officinalis*) Rosemary (*Rosmarinus officinalis*) Lemon balm (*Melissa officinalis*)	Clarifying
	Lavender (*Lavandula angustifolia*) Rose (*Rosa damascena*) Skullcap (*Scutellaria lateriflora*)	Soothing
	Rose geranium (*Pelargonium graveolens*) Chamomile (*Matricaria chamomilla*) Licorice root (*Glycyrrhiza glabra*)	Healing

Sun Protection

Sun protection is important, but it is also widely known that we live in a vitamin D–deficient society. Sunlight triggers the synthesis of vitamin D in the body, and we need vitamin D to help strengthen our bones. A little bit of sun exposure is beneficial for the skin, activating melanin, which acts as a natural protector from harmful UV rays. Sunshine also has antibacterial and antiseptic properties, and just 5 to 10 minutes a day has been shown to help counter breakouts.

All that being said, you do need sun protection. Too much UV exposure can burn the deeper layers of our skin. The effect of UV rays can also cause uneven pigmentation and age spots. Wear a hat, load up on internal anti-oxidants, and avoid the sun between the hours of 10 a.m. and 2 p.m.; depending on your region, this is generally when UV rays are the strongest. Brides should only use mineral sunscreens like zinc or titanium dioxide. Mineral sunscreens sit on top of the skin, reflecting UV rays, while chemical sunscreens disperse the UV rays in the body. Chemical sunscreens are inferior to mineral sunscreens because they contain smaller molecules, which penetrate into the bloodstream and can cause irritation. The chemicals in these sunscreens (including oxybenzone, avobenzone, octinoxate, octisalate, homosalate, and 4-methylbenzylidene camphor) have been linked to allergies and hormonal disruption—and the destruction of coral reefs. Also, be aware of silicones hiding in sunscreens.

They are often included to combat the tacky feeling of mineral ingredients. Silicones, typically dimethicone, are very pore-clogging. Be certain never to leave sunscreen in a hot car. The heat can change the composition of the ingredients and actually make your skin more sensitive to the sun!

Avoid sun exposure in the weeks leading up to your wedding. While it can be tempting to tan, it isn't worth it. You may very well end up burning your skin and ruining your wedding photos, and, even worse, end up with long-term harm. Sun damage can cause myriad problems, including premature aging and skin cancer. If you still want the look of a tan, a safer alternative would be to invest in a spray tan. The effects of a spray tan typically last a couple of weeks and look very natural when done by a trained professional. As with all treatments, trying this out months before your wedding will let you know how your skin will react. Look for a spray tan treatment containing no dihydroxyacetone, commonly referred to as DHA. DHA is an additive used for color and can cause damage to DNA. Exfoliate your whole body before the treatment, and avoid applying any lotions or oils beforehand. This will help the "tan" last longer and adhere more evenly. I would recommend getting this done at least 3 days before your wedding to make sure no spray tan rubs off onto your wedding dress.

Skin Care While Traveling

If you are traveling to a wedding destination, bridal shower, or honeymoon, pack all the products you have been using, including masks and spot treatments. Many skin-care lines sell travel kits, which make it easy and fun to bring everything along. Keep these miniature bottles to refill from your full-size products. If you can't find travel kits, purchase smaller bottles to refill. This will make it easier when traveling in the future, and you won't have to buy a whole new travel set next time you go out of town.

Build your own travel set:

- Body moisturizer
- Cleanser
- Eye moisturizer
- Face mask
- Facial balm
  (I use this on my
  hands, too!)
- Lip balm
- Moisturizer
- Serum (if needed)
- Spot treatment
- Sunscreen
- Toner

Traveling can be stressful on the body, and a routine will help you keep your sanity. If you're flying, increase your water consumption. In a plane, there is low humidity, which means water evaporates from the body quickly. Staying hydrated will also keep your immune system strong—the last thing you want is to be sick during your wedding! To support your skin on the outside, I always recommend packing a hydrating serum, mask, or balm and reapplying mid-flight to help combat dehydration.

SKIN-CARE ROUTINES
FOR YOUR FLIGHT

PREFLIGHT: Apply a hydrosol, hydrating serum or oil, eye treatment, and balm. The balm will be occlusive and seal all that moisture in while protecting your skin from the harsh elements of flying—use it for your face, lips, and hands. Do not forget your reusable water bottle and make an effort to drink up.

DURING THE FLIGHT: Drink a generous amount of water. I typically add about an extra 40 ounces [1.2 L] onto my usual intake and drink water whenever beverages are offered. Try to get an aisle seat because you should be making frequent trips to the bathroom. I also always pack electrolyte tablets, which are easy to drop into water.

ON A SHORT FLIGHT (LESS THAN 3 HOURS): Reapply balm at least once mid-flight. Do not forget your lips!

ON A LONG FLIGHT (LONGER THAN 3 HOURS): Reapply balm. A few hours into the flight, use a gentle cleanser, apply a 20-minute hydrating mask, and then repeat the preflight steps. Give yourself a facial massage while reapplying the balm. Light motions from the jawbone to collarbone will activate lymphatic flow.

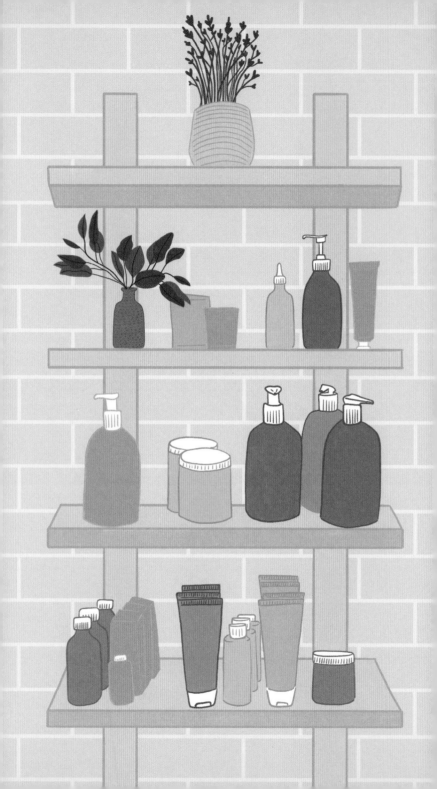

Ingredients to Avoid

Products are essentially designed to support your skin, but some ingredients and formulations can have adverse effects, such as clogged pores, dry skin, and much worse. There are various reasons these ingredients are included: to preserve the product, change the texture, hide a natural color, make the product smell nice, create a lather, strip away oils, and so on. While they do serve a purpose, they also work against the health of our skin. Particles can and do penetrate into the bloodstream and can harm our internal systems as well. The list of dangerous chemicals in the world of beauty is, unfortunately, long and tedious, but I've included an abbreviated list of common offenders below. If you find any of these in the products you have been using, it is time to phase them out. Safe replacements are making their debut every day!

Here are some common ingredients to avoid:

FRAGRANCE. When an ingredient list says "fragrance," that is a big red flag. It takes many ingredients to create an artificial scent, and formulators can conceal harmful, sometimes toxic, ingredients under this umbrella. Ingredients that have not been approved by the FDA can be snuck in this way.

SILICONES are nontoxic and create a wonderful glide and slippery feeling, so they are often used to alter texture. But of course, there is a price to pay. Silicone is a plastic-like substance that can get trapped deep in the pores, causing infection and blockages. Sometimes these effects are immediate, and sometimes they take years of daily use. They can also interfere with the skin's natural ability to create and retain moisture. Silicone ingredients typically end in "-cone." Dimethicone is the most common, found in everything from foundation to sunscreen.

PARABENS are common preservatives in cosmetic products. They are listed as butyl, methyl, ethyl, and propyl. Even though formulations typically use less than the legal 25 percent, even small amounts can be damaging. These ingredients mimic estrogen and have been linked to breast cancer and infertility.

SODIUM LAURYL SULFATE and **SODIUM LAURETH SULFATE** are foaming agents, more commonly found in toothpaste and shampoo. They can also creep into skin-care cleansers. Studies have linked these ingredients to cancer, neurotoxicity, organ toxicity, and endocrine disruption.

PHTHALATES are used in pesticides or to soften other ingredients, controlling the texture and making ingredients blend together nicely. While they may make a product feel super smooth, phthalates have been known to damage the reproductive organs, kidneys, and liver. The molecular size of phthalates makes them easy to absorb, and while they are usually expelled from the skin, buildup is hazardous. Using multiple products with phthalates can worsen the issue.

ALCOHOLS are tricky because not all alcohols dry and evaporate as one would think. Alcohols typically end in "-ol": ethanol, isopropyl alcohol, alcohol denat, methaol, benzyl, etc. If you are having issues with your skin, avoid them! They are used as solvents and preservatives in skin-care products and can cause breakouts and irritate skin.

Many of these ingredients are found not only in skincare, but makeup as well. If you're working with a makeup artist on your wedding day, ask if they can stick to natural products.

As a caveat on alcohols—cetearyl, stearyl, cetyl, and behenyl alcohol are fatty alcohols and can also be used as solvents. They can work to help hydrate the skin. These alcohols are typically used as emulsifiers, have little effect on the skin, and can actually help to bind moisture. For myself and my clients, I recommend only these types of alcohols, which are derived from organic whole plants: grapes, sugar cane, or grain.

When choosing safe alternatives, look for products with fewer ingredients in the list—the simpler, the better. If you are having a reaction to ingredients, and are not under the guidance of a professional, stick to a gentle cleanser, hydrosol, and simple oil until symptoms subside.

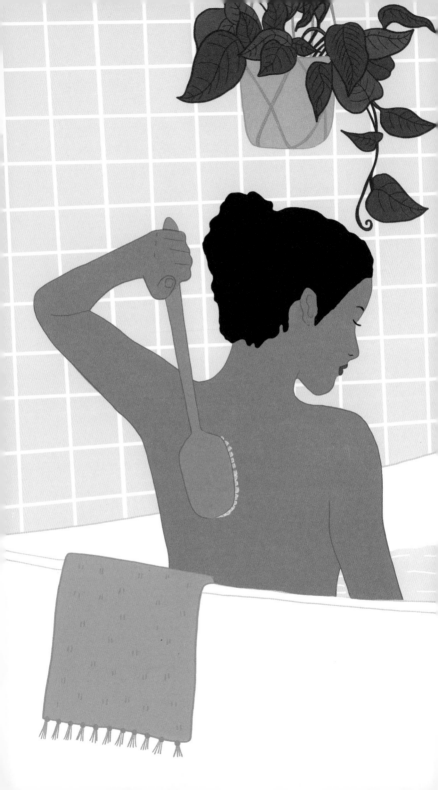

Caring for the Skin on Your Body

Be comfortable in your skin . . . all over! Glow is not just about the face, but the full body. You'll feel better and more vibrant knowing you have looked after all of your skin. Here are some tips for keeping the rest of your body smooth and radiant.

DRY BRUSHING

Dry brushing is one of my top recommendations for brides. Every time someone takes me up on the advice, I get rave reviews and disbelief in the results. Dry brushing touches on the integumentary (the system that includes hair, skin, nails, and exocrine glands), circulatory, and lymphatic systems. This routine softens skin, activates lymph flow, and can even out the texture of cellulite. The firm bristles physically remove any dry, dead surface skin cells, leaving you silky smooth and your skin more open for topical moisturizing treatments. The motions can activate lymphatic flow and assist in the detoxification of waste in the connective tissue of the skin by way of lymphatic drainage. Eliminating waste that is present in the tissues speeds up the metabolism of cellulite and smooths out the bumps and lumps it can cause. It is so simple, yet so effective.

Purchase a natural bristle brush—you can find these anywhere you find natural body products. Use the brush on dry skin, before showering or bathing. Make long, firm strokes up your limbs, toward your heart, and lighter, clockwise circles on the chest and stomach. Spending 1 to 3 minutes doing this before bathing can make a world of difference.

BODY WASH

Body washes can come in liquid, gels, creams, or bars. If you have a tendency toward drier skin, stick to a cream cleanser or a more hydrating bar. If your skin is well balanced, castile-based liquid soaps or hydrating soap bars are great. As always, watch out for toxic ingredients (see page 51). In liquid body washes, formulators love to include sulfates for a luxurious foam—not worth it! Bar soaps can overstrip and upset the skin's microbiome if they have harsh ingredients. Regardless of what soap you use, wash with natural fiber washcloths made from hemp or agave that have a rough texture for extra exfoliation.

SCRUBS

Like dry brushing, scrubs physically remove dry, dead surface skin cells. Look for scrubs with natural textures like oats, salt, or sugar. These leave the skin feeling silky smooth—and even hydrated if they contain an oil.

The thickest skin on our body is on the bottom of our feet. This skin can get dry and requires extra attention. To soften skin in this area, soak your feet for 5 minutes, then use a scrub with a pumice stone. This is a great ritual to indulge in the night before or day of your wedding. Following is an easy-to-assemble scrub for the body.

SIMPLE SCRUB

½ cup [120 ml] oil of your choice, such as melted coconut oil or olive oil

(If using coffee grounds, try not to let them go down the drain.)

½ cup [80 to 100 g] sugar, salt, oats, or coffee grounds

1 or 2 drops of your favorite essential oil

1. Mix the ingredients together and keep them in a container in the shower. Using your hands, scrub the mixture onto your body with motions toward the heart.

2. The scrub will last a week, and you should be able to get three or more uses from it.

MOISTURIZING

Body moisturizers should be applied after patting your skin dry, when it is still slightly dewy. This traps hydration against the skin. Like cleansing and exfoliating, how the body is moisturized depends on your skin's characteristics.

Almond oil or apricot oil are great, simple moisturizers for all skin types. You can buy them in bulk, in pure form, or with blends of other oils and herbal extracts. For drier skin, try an unscented or lightly scented butter. Raw shea butter or cocoa butter are my personal favorites. You can even melt raw, unrefined shea butter in a double boiler, add a drop or two of your favorite essential oil (no citrus—it can increase the risk of sunburn), and let solidify for a homemade, scented moisturizer.

Balms are beneficial for the driest areas, like the elbows, hands, and feet. They are a blend of wax and oils that have been heated, mixed, and cooled. Some contain herbal blends, and these can be particularly helpful for skin conditions such as psoriasis and eczema. A little goes a long way as they melt into the skin. Following is a balm recipe you can make at home to promote healing and hydration.

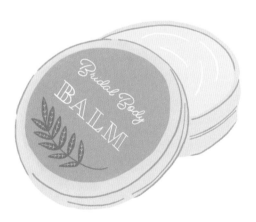

BRIDAL BODY BALM

5 oz [150 ml]
coconut oil

5 oz [150 ml]
olive oil

3 oz [90 ml]
beeswax

8 to 12 drops of
German chamomile
or rose essential oil

1 drop rosemary
extract (as a preser-
vative)

---

1. Make sure all equipment is clean and
    sanitized.

2. Warm coconut oil, olive oil, and beeswax
    in a double boiler or crockpot on low. Heat
    until the ingredients liquefy.

3. Let the mixture cool a few minutes, but
    don't let it solidify. Add essential oils and
    rosemary extract.

4. Pour into a jar or multiple shallow tins and
    allow to cool. Use when needed.

NOURISHING SKIN FROM THE INSIDE OUT

Nourishing the skin from the inside is just as important—if not more—than topical skin care. It is unlikely your skin will be and look healthy if your internal systems are suffering. The time leading up to the wedding is a great opportunity to support your body and all it does for you. It takes 30 days to create a habit and 28 days for cells to renew themselves. The earlier you start, the better the results. Do not forget to love your body—if you mindfully nourish yourself, you will feel better, look better, and glow better. This is the basis of holistic skin care.

Hydration

Hydration is a bride's best friend. We are made mostly of water, and water is necessary for every single cell in our bodies to function. Think of a cell as a water balloon. When the balloon is empty, it is deflated; it looks flat and folded. But when it is filled with water, it is smooth and plump, maintaining its shape. Studies have shown that 75 percent of Americans are chronically dehydrated. Visually, dehydration looks like "crepey" skin, having a granular texture. Hydrated skin is smoother in texture, and fine lines and wrinkles are less visible. Hydrated skin looks brighter and more youthful.

Dehydration not only causes fine lines and wrinkles to be more prominent. Other symptoms include headaches, dry mouth, muscle cramping, fatigue, foggy thinking, hunger, and of course . . . thirst! Look out for the signs and drink up. Your urine should be light in color to clear. In my personal experience, the more consistently I am hydrated, the less I have to think about it and the more my body will clue me in when it is time for a drink. As hydrating becomes more of a habit, it becomes easier to recognize when we are out of balance.

To reach full hydration takes an average of 3 days. You cannot binge drink water the day before your wedding and hope for the best. All this will do is flush out your minerals and cause frequent trips to the restroom, and it could cause serious illness if you really overdo it. So start now! The first step is finding a water bottle you love, preferably something made of glass, stainless steel, or ceramic. (The less plastic on the planet, the better.) Think of this bottle as an accessory, an extension of you, sticking with you throughout the day to help you reach all your glow goals.

Diuretics are the enemy of hydration. These are liquids that cause the expulsion of fluids from the body. They include alcohol and caffeinated drinks like coffee and tea. Diuretics are not necessarily bad, but they definitely work against your hydration efforts. If you're going to drink them, make sure to supplement with water and electrolytes. A good rule to adopt is when you drink a diuretic beverage, follow it up by drinking two glasses of water. This helps to offset the dehydration and avoid over-consumption.

Electrolytes replenish your body with vitamins and minerals. They are responsible for creating electric currents through the body. These electric currents are necessary for building new tissue, clotting the blood, balancing pH levels, and helping the functions of the muscles, nerves, and heart.

For example, sodium is an electrolyte necessary for balancing water content inside and outside the cells, especially in the blood, and an imbalance, either too much or too little, equals dehydration. Whether we're expelling too much, through natural elimination like urination and sweating, or ingesting too much, through processed foods that may contain high sodium, we need to bring sodium levels in our body back into balance.

Low-sugar electrolytes are a great supplementation and can counter an imbalance of sodium and assist in maintaining healthy hydration levels. They also typically contain potassium, calcium, magnesium, and sodium bicarbonate. They work wonders if you wake up feeling less than stellar after too much Champagne at your bachelorette party! For a daily boost of electrolytes, drink a glass of lemon water in the morning.

LOVE YOUR LYMPH TEA

1 tsp dried cleavers
(*Galium aparine*)

1 tsp echinacea
(*Echinacea purpurea*)

1 tsp dandelion
(*Taraxacum*)

¼ tsp licorice root
(*Glycyrrhiza glabra*), for sweetness and extra skin nourishment

1. Mix the dried herbs together and cover with 2 cups [120 ml] of boiling water.

2. Steep for 20 minutes.

3. Enjoy!

Lymphatic Drainage

The lymphatic system is the body's defense against diseases and infection. This network transports lymph, a fluid that contains infection-fighting white blood cells throughout the body, and also supports tissues by carrying away waste. Our lymphatic system is a large part of building and maintaining our immunity. This hardworking network is constantly cleansing the blood and fluid in our tissues, and returning it to the heart as clean blood. This detoxification process by way of the lymphatic system is really what creates our inner and outer glow.

You can picture this system as a network of rivers, waterfalls, and pools lying just under the skin. Water is drained into the system through even smaller runoffs in tissues throughout the body. The pools are where waste is filtered out and carried away in another direction. Clean, flowing water results in skin that radiates wellness. Put another way, as one of my favorite fellow holistic estheticians, Angela Peck, says, "No flow, no glow."

Our blood pressure and muscle contractions determine the speed of lymph movement, but we can accelerate the process with professional manual lymph treatments or at-home treatments such as dry brushing (see page 55) and gua sha (see page 66).

Drinking water will also encourage lymphatic movement, as will lymphatic herbs. You can support your lymphatic system with tinctures or teas like the one here (facing page).

Gua Sha

Gua sha is an ancient Chinese facial rejuvenation therapy that assists in regenerating tissues, moving stagnant lymph, and breaking up muscle tension. A smooth-edged gua sha tool is used to glide across oiled skin to stimulate micro-circulation within the skin. These tools for gua sha come in different shapes and are made of various materials: porcelain, stainless steel, and crystals like rose quartz and jade. In traditional Chinese medicine, these tools are used to move qi (pronounced "chi"), which means life-force energy, throughout the body. Qi is necessary for vitality and strength, and its circulation is considered an important way to increase those properties. This practice creates movement in the tissues, activating cells to receive nutrients and detoxify, which, in turn, reduces

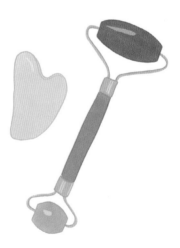

puffiness, calms inflammation, lightens dark circles, eases hyperpigmentation, and decreases redness.

A gua sha routine can be 1 to 25 minutes long. It is a relaxing form of facial massage that shows instant results. Here's a simple routine that can be done daily.

Using a gua sha tool, glide the scraper with light to medium pressure up and down the neck, and then work upward (starting at the chin and working toward the forehead) with long strokes from the center of your face and out. Finish with long strokes on the sides of the face, down the neck, and to the collarbone.

A few notes before you get started: Gua sha is not a good idea if you have a tendency to get broken capillaries. Do it with light pressure, so as not to create a lasting redness or bruising. Tools can be found at crystal stores, herbal shops, your esthetician's office, or online (refer to resources in the back of this book). When purchasing crystals, please make sure they are from a reputable source. Jade rollers can be used in a similar way to create some circulation and lymphatic flow but will not have quite the same effects as gua sha. Gua sha goes a little deeper, covers more surface area, and soothes more muscle tension. With either a gua sha tool or a jade roller, use a generous amount of facial oil of your choosing beforehand. You want there to be a light glide on the skin versus a drag.

Exercise

A regular exercise routine is key to maintaining glow. Moving your body elevates your heart rate, increasing blood flow. Increased blood flow means more oxygen in the blood and more nourishment to the cells working through your body. Regular exercise promotes healthy cell growth, supports collagen and elastin, improves muscle tone, and physically creates thicker, more supple skin. A healthy, balanced regimen will help to balance hormones. When hormones are more in balance, you will have fewer breakouts and monthly menstrual-related breakouts, as the stress hormone cortisol is kept in check.

Think of exercise as the gift that keeps on giving. You give yourself the time for movement, and in return, it gives you balance, not to mention all of those endorphins that feel so good.

When preparing for my wedding, I thoroughly appreciated my workout routine. It was time devoted to only caring for my body, and I would always finish feeling stronger and refreshed. If you are new to exercising, start slow and be realistic with yourself. Find something that is convenient, fun, and challenging. It's a good idea to switch up your routine to use different muscles and avoid plateau. If you usually run, why not try rock climbing to strengthen your arms? Or, if you like to cycle, try yoga to stretch out your leg muscles and limber up.

Allow yourself space for recovery, and be sure not to overdo it! It is essential to rest after a workout to repair muscles. Over-exercising or exercising without proper nutrition can work against your health and wellness. A personal trainer can be a great guide in this process of getting started. Before establishing an exercise routine, be sure to consult with your doctor.

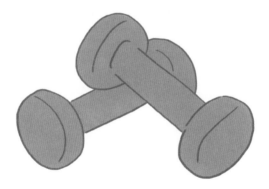

Diet

Skin health, and health in general, is directly related to what we put into our bodies. How we feed our body determines the health of our cells, so eat with the intention to nourish. Our bodies and what they need vary, and this can change over time, but we all need a balanced diet of clean proteins, healthy fats, antioxidant-rich whole foods, and an array of nutrients such as beta carotene, vitamins C and E, zinc, and selenium.

Skin-care supplements are sold to streamline the process of absorbing different nutrients. Supplements are great, although they vary in quality. When thoughtfully eating a balanced diet, you should be able to get your daily intake of vitamins through your food. Consult with a doctor or nutritionist before taking any supplements.

Here are the vitamins and minerals that you should prioritize in the lead-up to your wedding (and beyond!) to achieve a balanced, wholesome diet and maximum glow.

ANTIOXIDANTS defend cells from free radicals. Free radicals are molecules that have an uneven number of electrons, and therefore steal electrons from healthy cells in our body, creating an imbalance. They oxidize healthy cells, essentially destroying or damaging cell membranes, speeding up the process of aging and stealing your glow. Eating antioxidant-rich foods is a good way to internally protect your skin from the sun. They will not take the place of sunscreen but can help in both preventing sun damage and repairing the effects of UV rays.

Here are some antioxidant-rich foods that will help prevent sun and general tissue damage. (These are not intended to take the place of sun protection, but rather to be used as an aid!)

- Artichokes
- Beets
- Black beans
- Blackberries
- Blueberries
- Broccoli
- Cloves
- Coffee
- Goji berries

- Grapes
- Green Tea
- Kale
- Peaches
- Pecans
- Red cabbage
- Strawberries
- Walnuts
- Yellow and red peppers

CAROTENOIDS also deliver high amounts of antioxidants and promote healthy cell growth. Provitamin A carotenoids, such as beta-carotene, will convert to vitamin A, which helps to maintain healthy skin by strengthening and replacing skin cells. Benefits of carotenoids include increasing the skin's ability to maintain hydration, more evened skin tone, and reduction in inflammation. Fruits and vegetables that are red, orange, and yellow carry high levels of carotenoids. Carotene is the pigment that colors these plants. When cartenoids are paired with other foods, they increase the bioavailability of other nutrients, as well.

COLLAGEN is a protein which gives the skin its form and structure. Collagen is beneficial for helping to maintain the health of skin, as well as improving tone and texture. I prefer plant-based alternatives to support collagen function, including foods or supplements high in zinc and vitamin C, which are necessary for collagen production. The snow ear mushroom works as a great substitute for animal-derived collagen.

HEALTHY FATS are delicious and are needed for reducing inflammatory responses and protecting your skin from harmful UV rays. Some fatty, rich foods that will lend to your glow are avocados, Brazil nuts, coconuts and coconut oil, and olives and olive oil.

Omega-3 and omega-6 fatty acids are essential to combating aging and to healing and repairing the skin. They also assist in managing oil production, proving to be helpful for acne. These essential fatty acids can be sourced from flax seeds, walnuts, chia seeds, and fish. The delicious smoothie recipe on the facing page is full of antioxidants and fatty acids.

Digestive triggers are foods that set your digestive system off, causing inflammation or bloating and possibly a skin disturbance. The main triggers are gluten, dairy, sugar, alcohol, and processed foods. I see so many people who completely change their skin by eliminating one element of their diet. Doing this requires full removal of the suspected food from all meals. If you are not feeling well, or are concerned about receiving proper nutrition, please consult a nutritionist. Sometimes it can be obvious what needs to be cut out; other times it is more ambiguous. Signs of dietary intolerances are persistent breakouts, bloating, indigestion, acid reflux, constipation, diarrhea, irritability, etc.

We all have an emotional relationship with food. The idea of eliminating foods that you have eaten your entire life can be very daunting. People with a history of eating disorders should consult with a nutritionist or doctor before cutting

SKIN-HEALTHY SMOOTHIE

1 cup [240 ml] organic almond milk

½ cup [60 g] strawberries

¼ cup [35 g] blueberries

½ banana

1 Tbsp ground flaxseed

½ tsp matcha powder

1. Toss the ingredients in a blender and mix until smooth.

2. Enjoy!

SKIN ESSENTIAL	SOURCES
Vitamin A (*retinol*)	Leafy green vegetables, like kale and spinach; yellow, orange, and red fruits and vegetables; yams
B vitamins	Beans, whole grains, avocados, bananas, seeds, and nuts
Vitamin C (*ascorbic acid*)	Citrus fruits, broccoli, Brussels sprouts, strawberries and other berries
Vitamin D	Sunlight, mushrooms, fortified drinks, like orange juice or almond milk
Vitamin E (*tocopherol*)	Nuts, whole grains, leafy green vegetables
Vitamin K	Leafy green vegetables, whole grains, vegetable oils, cruciferous vegetables like broccoli and cauliflower
Vitamin P (*bioflavonoids*)	Most fruits and vegetables, especially those richer in color, like cherries, blueberries, tomatoes, and green peppers
Calcium	Seeds, green vegetables, cabbage, okra, molasses
Sodium	Sodium is salt and should be used in moderation; beets and celery have a natural sodium content
Zinc	Whole grains, nuts, seeds, and legumes, like garbanzo beans and lentils

HOW IT HELPS

Aids in cellular function and strength, promotes elasticity, and both prevents and reverses sun damage.

B vitamins should be taken as a complex since there are various types. They work synergistically to promote metabolism. They also support integumentary tissues (hair, skin, nails) and functions of the nervous system, and they prevent oxidative stress.

Powerful antioxidant, builds healthy cell walls to prevent broken capillaries and bruising.

Promotes healthy healing of the skin's tissues. Helps our body maintain and use calcium.

A powerful antioxidant preventing tissue damage throughout the body.

Strengthens capillary walls and aids in blood clotting.

Enhances the absorption of vitamin C, assists in building healthy cells, acts as an antioxidant, and supports healthy blood circulation.

Aids in healthy barrier function of the skin and helps skin achieve homeo-stasis.

Maintains carbon dioxide and water levels in the cells. Helps muscle, nerve, and digestion function.

Improves collagen production and strengthens the immune system.

anything out of their diet. If you are eliminating a trigger, focusing on what you *can* eat, instead of what you *cannot*, is helpful. Having healthy alternatives on hand will help in setting yourself up for success. If it becomes obvious that a food is a trigger, it will make it easier to abstain. Ideally, you should cut something out for at least four weeks; however, you may see improvements to confirm you are on the right track much earlier. If you think you may have a dietary trigger that is affecting your skin health, try eliminating food groups from your diet now, so you can identify any issues long before your wedding.

Good digestion is essential for healthy skin, but it is not only *what* you are eating; it is also *how* you are eating. If you are stressed or anxious *while* you are eating, or you don't take the time to fully chew as you eat, food does not get broken down and absorbed correctly. This faulty digestion can cause major issues later in the digestive process. Conscious eating helps our bodies absorb nutrients and digest more easily. If we are taking the time to sit and eat, to actually look at our food and chew it thoroughly, our digestive system is creating the necessary secretions to break down our food. Eating mindfully puts less stress on the gut. Happy gut means happy skin.

A SAMPLE DAY OF
SKIN-HEALTHY MEALS

BREAKFAST

Skin-Healthy Smoothie (see recipe on
page 73) or oatmeal with chia seeds,
blueberries, and raspberries

MORNING SNACK

Handful of cashews or a piece of fruit

LUNCH

Vegetable curry with rice or a smoked tempeh
sandwich with lettuce and tomato

AFTERNOON SNACK

Seaweed snacks or nut butter and celery

DINNER

Lentil soup or a protein of your choice (beans
and rice, lentils, tofu, fish, etc.) and kale salad
with Amino Acid Dressing (mix together 1 part
Bragg Liquid Aminos, 1 part lemon juice,
1 part olive oil)

SOMETHING SWEET

Avocado chocolate mousse or frozen mangos
and strawberries

Sleep

The whole concept of beauty sleep is real. Missing a full night of rest can leave you feeling less than your best, and your skin will show it, too. Puffiness or dark circles are some of the common symptoms of lack of sleep, but not getting enough sleep can also increase the appearance of fine lines and wrinkles. REM sleep allows our body to repair itself at night. Essential tissue repair happens while we sleep or rest. During this time, our liver is hard at work preparing itself with energy for the next day.

To better understand how important rest is, it helps to understand the two nervous system states, the **PARASYM-PATHETIC** and the **SYMPATHETIC**. Sympathetic is the "fight or flight or freeze" response. This is the state your entire body is in when your body is called to action. Think of an anxiety attack as the extreme of this state, or being stalked by a hunting lion. This state is what gets us out of bed in the morning—think adrenaline, cortisol, etc. It is necessary for us to be alert and to function. However, too much time spent in this state can harm and deplete our bodies.

Parasympathetic is the "rest and digest" state. This is our body's time to repair tissues, digest to distribute energy, and rest for the next sympathetic response. The extreme of this state would be transcendental meditation, sleep, or, to use a different lion analogy, when the lion is sleeping for days, digesting its food, and preparing for the next hunt. It is important to tap into this state as much as possible, to train our body to repair itself and not get caught up in the sympathetic state, which can cause insomnia, general inflammation, and premature aging. The parasympathetic nervous system is when your body is calm, suppressing high energy, and taking time to repair itself. This is when tissues mend, heal, and can be rejuvenated.

Nightly routines are a signal to your body that it is time to wind down. A mindful nighttime skin-care ritual can help ease into your bridal beauty sleep. Going to bed and waking up at the same time each morning stamps a sleep routine into your internal clock. Brides should aim for 8 hours of sleep. Count back 8 hours from the time you need to wake up. And don't forget to leave time for your nighttime skin-care rituals before turning out the lights.

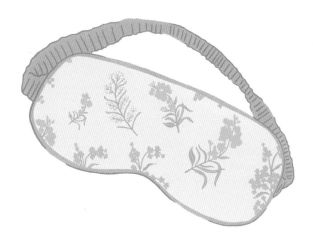

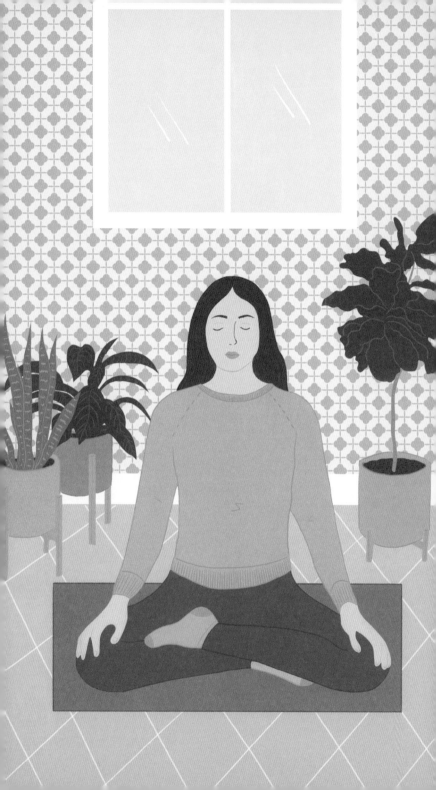

Stress Management

Preparing for a wedding can be so fun, but as a bride, you may be putting a lot of stress on yourself. All the planning, tasks, decisions, and opinions can really add up—not to mention all these systems you are putting in place to take care of yourself. Stress wreaks havoc on every system in our body, including our skin. It spikes our cortisol levels and drains our adrenals. Adrenals are glands that produce hormones, more specifically stress hormones. When we are constantly stressed, these glands can be drained and cause loss of energy. Their supply can be rebuilt by managing stress. It only makes sense that internal stress shows up outwardly through our body's largest organ. Here are some ways to support yourself and manage your stress levels during this time—because managed stress means glowing skin.

MEDITATION is a great tool for tapping into the parasympathetic nervous state. The effects include feelings of calm, grounding, and the ability to cope with daily stresses. It takes practice and gets easier the more you do it. Guided meditation or classes can be very helpful. Before my wedding, I meditated solo, and I also used float tanks. These are often called sensory deprivation tanks, and they work by closing you off from all stimuli as you submerge yourself in water and enough Epsom salt to float and feel weightless. It gave me a sense of calm, renewing my energy and helping me sleep. I did this once a week and would leave feeling cleansed and stress free.

De-stressing does not always have to be solo! Studies show that **SOCIALIZING** elevates dopamine and builds the confidence that enables us to cope more easily with external stressors. It is helpful to bounce ideas off people and vent, if needed. Invite friends and family along on wedding planning excursions.

GO OUTSIDE. Take a walk, hike, sail a boat, get outside and do whatever you enjoy! Being outside and breathing in negative ion–filled oxygen has a positive impact on our bodies and initiates a calming feeling. And sunshine can help, too. Vitamin D not only supports bone health but has been linked to a decrease in both depression and general inflammation. Just be careful when taking in those UV rays and use protection!

Book some of the **TREATMENTS** listed in the section beginning on page 87. Try anything and everything that appeals to you. All will initiate an inner peace and centered mindset to help you take on wedding planning. And, as an added bonus, these treatments will help you visibly glow! Scheduling time for self-care is essential.

If you are feeling particularly stressed, taking herbs can help alleviate emotional burden. Adaptogens help to balance cortisol levels and strengthen the body's ability to cope with stress. Some common adaptogenic herbs are ashwagandha, rhodiola, lion's mane, and ginseng. CBD, the major constituent in the Cannabis plant, is also a great tool for neutralizing anxious feelings. CBD is short for cannabidiol, a molecule which collaborates with our endocannabinoid system. Hemp-derived CBD is non-psychoactive, unlike its cousin THC, and creates a sense of tranquility for most people. Herbal remedies in tincture form are a simple method of delivery, as they are easy to take in a dropper under the tongue. Teas and capsules are easy methods as well. Please make sure that you are purchasing high quality products and check with your doctor before use. Here is an easy herbal tea for stress reduction.

DE-STRESS TEA

½ tsp lemon balm   ½ tsp peppermint

½ tsp skullcap   ½ tsp ashwagandha

1. Mix the ingredients together in a mug and cover with boiling water.

2. Let steep for 10 to 20 minutes.

3. Drink and breathe deeply.

WEDDING TIMELINE

On the subject of scheduling, coming up with a timeline for wedding planning is crucial and can help you learn to manage stress in the future. Start immediately so you can relax and glow when you get closer to the date. Be realistic and do not forget to ask for help when needed. Stop and savor every step.

Everyone's bridal glow journey looks a bit different, but a typical wedding timeline might look something like the following.

A self-care mantra that has stuck with me is "Be kind to your future self." Establishing a plan and taking care of business now will save you a headache later on!

1 YEAR BEFORE

Find an esthetician and establish a skin-care routine with products you love.

10 MONTHS BEFORE

Try whatever treatments you are drawn to or are appropriate for your skin type. Establish an exercise routine and think about whether your diet may be impacting your skin.

6 MONTHS BEFORE

Six months out is the latest you should start testing out any treatments that may be beneficial before the wedding, like a spray tan or body scrub. This is also a good time to start any treatments that you want to repeat in the run up to the big day, like facials.

2 WEEKS TO 2 DAYS BEFORE

Get a massage and facial.

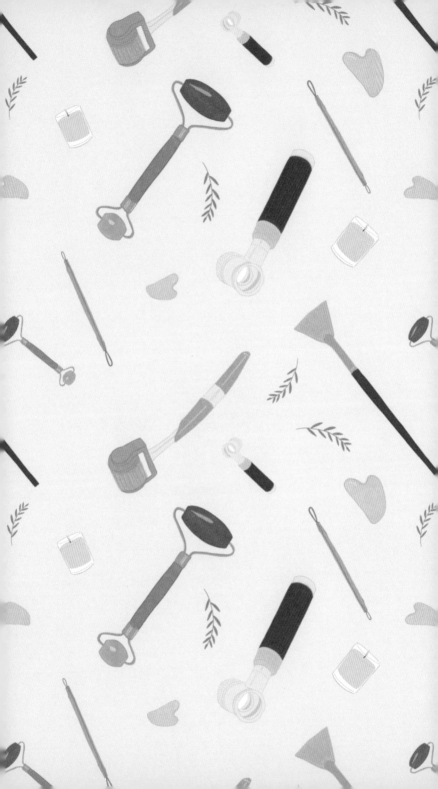

PROFESSIONAL TREATMENTS

The time leading up to your wedding is a time to pamper yourself. Take time to rest, recover, and . . . get a treatment! Treatments can make you feel better in your skin and are a great time out from all the wedding planning. A spa treatment should help relax you and tap into the parasympathetic nervous system. There are many different types of professional skin-care treatments: for the body or for the face, invasive or gentle. Start engaging with an esthetician as soon as possible! I cannot stress this enough. The sooner, the better. Brides who seek new treatments a week or even a month before their wedding are taking a risk of having a bad reaction close to their wedding date. Don't be that bride.

Choosing an Esthetician

For taking care of facial skin, a facial from an esthetician is a great place to start. I sometimes describe a facial as "a more productive massage." There are plenty of benefits to massage: relaxation, improved circulation (i.e., oxygen and blood flow), more flexibility, better recovery, and a stronger immune system. With a facial, you walk out with similar rewards—plus, some education on caring for your newly glowing skin. A good facial treatment will provide you with deep exfoliation, jump-start your cellular turn-over, and treat ailments. Ideally, you will also learn how to improve your complexion with an at-home routine. This will provide a solid base for glowing on your wedding day. Your esthetician may also provide treatments to help with the skin on your back or décolletage to help you look your best in your wedding dress.

There are a variety of different esthetician styles and approaches. Treatments can range from very straight-forward and clinical to the most relaxing, dreamy experience ever.

I recommend a holistic esthetician who uses natural, plant-based products. Estheticians who call themselves holistic should have an understanding of the different systems of the body and how they support one another. Holistic estheticians may also identify themselves as being "natural," "organic," "green," etc. Fortunately, the popularity of the holistic esthetician field is growing; a quick online search will show you who is available in your area.

If you are already using a professional product line you love or come across one in your search, look for a "Stockists" button on the company's website, which will list the estheticians who use that brand.

Once you've identified a few local estheticians, check out their websites. Are you attracted to one over the other? This is an intimate service, so it is important to choose someone you feel comfortable with. No holistic esthetician in the area? Look for an esthetician who uses a cleaner product line. Oftentimes, estheticians will carry an organic line in addition to a more conventional line.

To initialize a rapport, you can start by sending an email or giving them a call. Inform your esthetician of what you are looking for and your wedding date. If you have any specific concerns or goals, or if you are looking for a new skin-care regimen in general, this is a good time to discuss that as well.

Try to get your first treatment at least six months prior to your wedding; a year is even better. You will see results after one facial, but the effects are compounding and can only get better with each treatment. This does not mean you have to get facials every month until your wedding. You and your esthetician can set guidelines and create a customized plan that works for you, taking both your budget and timeline into account. A little planning and booking appointments well in advance can prevent a lot of stress in the long run.

Things to Know Before You Go

There is not much preparation that needs to take place, but here are some tips to make the most of your time and to make sure you do not compromise your skin before your treatment.

- Think about your skin goals. What would you like to achieve long term? What do you love about your skin? What areas would you like to improve?

- Share your skin-care goals, wedding date, and what you would like to achieve before the wedding day. This will help your esthetician direct you regarding timeline, products, routines, and more.

- Avoid too much sun exposure before your appointment. A sunburn will inflame your skin, and your esthetician will be forced to focus on healing your skin rather than treating your concerns. If the burn is bad enough, they may turn you away altogether.

- Avoid strong exfoliation before your treatment. No concentrated acids, enzymes, or vitamin A (retinol) products. Using these products within 3 days of your appointment can increase your chances of having a reaction.

- Take photos of the ingredient lists on your skin-care products, or at the very least bring the names of your products. Oftentimes, the ingredients are only listed on the box, but sometimes they can be found online. Having the names and ingredient lists on hand will be helpful for an esthetician when they ask you what you are using. This gives your new esthetician a solid baseline of what your skin can handle, what it responds well to, any red flags that may need to be addressed, and so on.

- Let your esthetician know if you have a history of reactions to products. Also, be prepared to list any medical conditions or medications you are taking. Sometimes there are contraindications, and the treatment will need to be altered. Make it known if you are pregnant, breastfeeding, or trying to conceive.

- Consider your current skin-care routine. Think about how much you want to invest in at-home skin care. Treatments are so effective, but without the correct daily support, you may be undoing everything that was accomplished in the facial treatment. Having a budget in mind, or knowing which products you want to replace or keep, can help you feel prepared when talking with your esthetician.

- Do not worry about washing your face before your facial. Your esthetician will do a thorough cleansing and take off anything that needs to be removed. That being said, please do not put on a full face of makeup for your appointment. If you arrive with a lot of makeup, the removal will inevitably cut into the treatment time of your facial.

- Hydration is important for general skin health, so hopefully you are drinking your water! Be sure to use the restroom before your facial. There's nothing worse than trying to relax while needing to pee! Avoid drinking coffee or tea before your service.

- Be prepared to undress. You will not be fully exposed, since it is a facial treatment. Your esthetician may provide a robe, or have you lie under some sheets.

- Relax! Or rather, get ready to relax. Make sure you do not have big plans or an event immediately following your facial treatment. Your skin may be flushed and it's best not to apply makeup to freshly exfoliated skin. Plus, you may feel too blissed out to get much done.

During Your Treatment

No two facials are alike. Facials are customized for every-one's unique skin type, concerns, and wedding glow goals. Here are some things to expect, but really, as long as you are lying down, there is nothing you can do wrong!

- Take some deep breaths. You have nowhere else to be for an hour or so.

- Feel free to ask questions, but refrain from being too chatty—this is your time to relax your nervous system. However, if you are excited and feeling curious, or really itching to get to know your esthetician, have at it. This is a judgment-free zone. Just be sure to set aside some time for enjoying the quiet. Activating the parasympathetic nervous system is key to "rest and digest"—tapping into this as much as possible will help you achieve your skin-care goals faster.

- Facial treatments vary greatly, but your treatment should involve a form of cleansing, an analysis of your skin state, exfoliation, massage, and a healing mask. The process should also include an explana-tion of what your esthetician is seeing, what can be improved, and what the treatment will entail.

- If your esthetician finds it necessary, they will perform extractions—manually express your pores. This can be uncomfortable, especially on the nose. Just know it will be over quickly and is not a lasting pain.

- The esthetician will look at your skin under a bright light and magnifying glass. During this time, your esthetician is assessing your skin—red flags, issues that need to be addressed, or areas that need to be avoided. What you need may be different with each visit.

- By the time you have your last visit before the wedding, your esthetician will have a good idea of what works best for your skin. At the end of the entire process, you should feel like you have learned about your skin, how to better care for it, and how to achieve maximum glow on your wedding day.

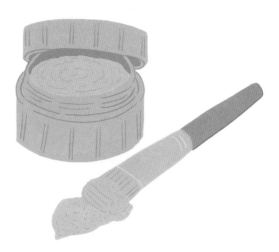

After Your Treatment

After a facial treatment, your skin is freshly exfoliated and exposed in a way that it wasn't before. Dead surface skin cells have been removed and your pores have been opened, leaving skin more vulnerable. Here are a few tips to consider after your treatment.

- Go about your typical routine, avoiding exfoliants for 48 hours, unless your esthetician guides you otherwise.

- Avoid makeup immediately after leaving. Your pores are open, so depending on the ingredients in your products, makeup application can cause irritation or breakouts. It is best to simply avoid altogether.

- Limit sun exposure immediately after leaving. Your freshly exfoliated skin may be more photosensitive.

- Your esthetician may have given you some instructions. Follow them. Pay attention to when your skin looks its best. Is it 3 days after your facial? Five days? This can help determine when it's best to schedule your pre-wedding treatment.

- If your skin has a negative reaction . . . stay calm. Contact your esthetician, send photos, and let them know what is going on. They may know exactly what happened, invite you back for a remedy, advise you to take an over-the-counter antihistamine, or refer you to a trusted dermatologist. It is *very* rare, but it happens from time to time. Reactions typically calm down as quickly as they start. Using new skin care is like eating a new food: There is a small chance your body will not agree with it. Let your esthetician know what has happened so they can help you.

• Schedule your follow up treatments!

SAMPLE FACIAL TREATMENT TIMELINE

1 YEAR BEFORE THE WEDDING

Schedule monthly to quarterly facials after your first visit to the esthetician, and establish a working skin-care routine.

6 MONTHS TO ONE MONTH BEFORE

Prioritize a monthly facial (if recommended by your esthetician).

1 MONTH BEFORE

Schedule one facial treatment, as recommended by your esthetician.

1 WEEK BEFORE

Schedule one facial treatment.

Other Facial Treatments to Consider

In the run-up to your wedding, you may want to consider other facial treatments, such as peels or microderm-abrasion. Some of these treatments can be done during a standard facial by an esthetician, while others should be performed only by dermatologists or doctors. Who can do what treatment varies from state to state. Some of these treatments have watered-down, at-home versions; however, I recommend professional guidance as oftentimes the DIY versions stray far from the original treatment.

PEELS are specialized treatments performed by a licensed professional using a measured percentage of acid. They promise a more even skin tone and texture, dimin-ished lines and wrinkles, lessened acne scarring, and a clear complexion. Peels lower the pH of the skin and remove dead surface skin cells and the "glue" that keeps them on the skin. Some peels are mild, leaving no immediate visible effect; others are deep and can cause an intense burning and then redness or peeling skin for days after. I do not recommend any peel that requires "downtime" (peeling, redness). Skin can be unpredictable with reactions to peels, as inflammation is inevitable, but I would never rec-ommend achieving these extreme aftereffects as a goal. Peels that do this are essentially creating an open wound, temporarily leaving the skin more vulnerable to environ-mental damage. I believe there is a time and a place for peels, but as with any sort of exfoliation, they should be done in moderation and with caution—over-exfoliation can age skin, breaking down the skin's ability to repair itself. Some at-home products are marketed as "peels," and although the acid percentage is lower than the peels used professionally, acids should be used under supervision. Consult your esthetician.

MICRODERMABRASION is a form of physical exfoliation involving a vacuum and then a form of exfoliation, either a "diamond-tip" grit surrounding the vacuum, sodium bicarbonate crystals, or acids. The goal of microdermabrasion is to exfoliate the skin, evening out skin tone and texture; it is often used to repair acne scarring. Microdermabrasion should never be done when redness or broken capillaries are present. Just like peels, microdermabrasion has a time and a place, but it should be used with caution. Inflamed, red skin should not be the goal. Using a vacuum on the skin can be dangerous and break capillaries, spread bacteria, and aggravate present skin issues.

Acupuncture is widely known, but have you ever considered an **ACUPUNCTURE FACIAL**? This treatment is a part of traditional Chinese medicine and involves an acupuncturist carefully and intentionally inserting tiny, tiny needles into specific points in the face. The needles used for facial treatments are typically smaller than those used on the body, minimizing or even eliminating any discomfort you may feel. In fact they are so small you often do not even feel them, and it is actually very relaxing and healing. These facials stimulate collagen and relax the facial muscles that tense up and lead to fine lines and wrinkles. This practice can leave the skin firmer and brighter for your wedding day. A session lasts 45 minutes to 1 hour and leads to deep relaxation. Acupuncture facials are great for all sorts of conditions, both physical and mental, and work best as a series. Your acupuncturist can help determine how many visits will be needed to achieve desired results.

MICROCURRENT facials stimulate collagen and elastin by emitting a low voltage electrical current through two nodes and into the body. Originally created to treat symptoms of Bell's palsy, it can be used to lift and tone facial muscles. A microcurrent facial could be a great short-term treatment to lift and tone, especially during the week or days leading up to a wedding, but I am skeptical of the long-term effects of putting a simulated electrical current through the body.

GUA SHA performed by a trained professional can be a very beneficial treatment. Refer to page 66 for more information. This is a great way to accomplish glow, and I highly recommend seeking out a professional treatment before attempting an at-home gua sha massage. This should not be performed on active breakouts or open skin.

FACIAL CUPPING provides many of the same benefits as gua sha. This practice involves dragging a cup and creating suction on the skin, causing the relaxation of muscle tension, stimulation of blood, and initiation of lymph movement. Results include a brighter complexion, toned muscles, and a decrease in puffiness. At-home facial cups are available, but to avoid broken capillaries and bruising, this is best done by a professional.

MICRONEEDLING involves short, small needles rolled over the skin. It creates a micro-trauma to the skin and activates new cell growth and collagen production. People experience smoother skin texture and more even skin tone. I would only recommend this procedure for localized areas and for treating deep, pitted scarring. Any time you introduce a trauma to the skin by puncturing it, you are weakening its natural strength, and over time this can cause premature aging.

MANUAL LYMPHATIC DRAINAGE is systematically manipulating and activating the lymphatic system, initiating detoxification and the flow of nutrients throughout the tissues of the skin (and the rest of the body). This treatment is a series of technical, often featherweight pulses that may not feel like they are doing much. It is a light, relaxing treatment that should only be carried out by a trained professional. Gua sha is a great, safe way to activate lymph flow at home. Benefits include brighter, more toned skin, healthier complexion, and reduction in any swelling.

LED THERAPY, or light-emitting diode therapy, involves a panel, wand, or mask that emits different wavelengths of light for different skin conditions. Indications for this noninvasive procedure are rosacea, acne, wrinkles, hyperpigmentation, and scarring. This treatment can be done at various strengths, sometimes requiring a recovery period to reduce inflammation. I think LED is a great option when other avenues have been exhausted.

There are some treatment options that are generally not a good idea:

HYDRAFACIALS use a vacuum to cleanse and exfoliate the skin, then infuse the skin with targeted hydrating serums. This treatment's goal is to leave the skin feeling hydrated and plump; some even claim to perform extractions. I have yet to see a hydrafacial that infuses anything worth penetrating into the skin. Again, vacuums can be harmful to the structure and function of the skin.

DERMAPLANING involves gliding a blade over the skin, exfoliating dead surface skin cells and removing the fine, vellus hair—or peach fuzz—on the face. People enjoy the smoothing effects and the way makeup glides on afterward. It also causes an inflammation and swelling that can temporarily reduce the appearance of fine lines and wrinkles. I do not recommend dermaplaning or shaving to remove peach fuzz. Doing so disrupts the barrier function of the skin and can cause sensitivity. Plus, vellus hair grows back blunt, creating a rough texture that is more noticeable. If you have face or body hair that you want to remove, waxing or sugaring are great alternatives to dermaplaning and other kinds of shaving.

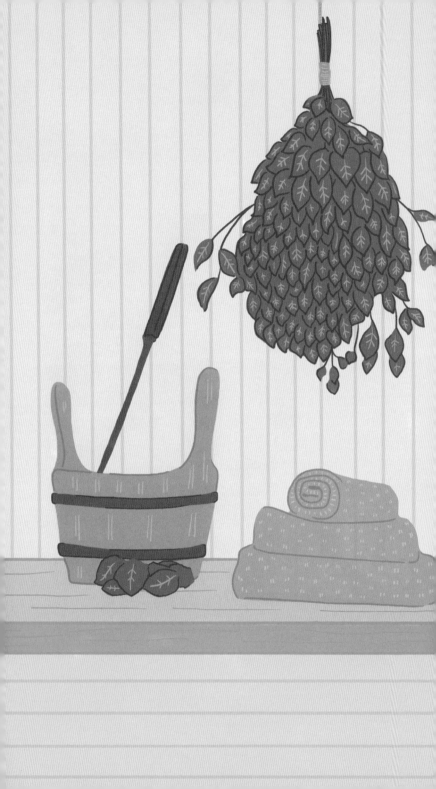

Body Treatments

Body treatments can encourage deep relaxation, stress management, and great skin, all of which are important when preparing for your wedding. The following treatments assist in achieving glow, and each has an extensive list of benefits—not all of which are listed here. Any of these treatments would be great the week, or even day, of your wedding. Whichever treatments you choose, be certain to test them before the month leading up to your wedding. Chances of having a reaction are slim, but it's best not to put yourself at risk.

SKIN SCRUBS involve lying down nude, or mostly nude, and having your body (excluding the face) manually scrubbed with salt or sugar. This activates lymph flow and physically removes dead surface skin cells. These therapies will leave you feeling smooth and rejuvenated, and they are wonderful for a quick, all-over body glow. These services range from very relaxing to almost painful, depending on the type of spa you visit. A skin scrub can be done right before the wedding date, or multiple times before.

THERMAL WRAPS raise your blood temperature while your body is wrapped in mud, seaweed, salt, or oils. This results in a detoxifying effect, drawing out sweat and, with it, toxins. Sometimes thermal wraps are accompanied by a scrub. Assisting the body in detoxifying leads to healthy, cleansed tissues and skin to give your body extra glow for the big day.

A **MUD BATH** is just what it sounds like, a mixture of mud and clay in which you submerge yourself. The mud in a mud bath is mineral-rich, often filled with potassium and magnesium, which are known to calm muscles and soften the skin. Note that mud baths are not for the claustrophobic. This treatment is super luxurious and is great for a bride who wants to feel pampered. (And who doesn't?)

SAUNAS raise your core temperature and activate heat-stress proteins, in turn strengthening your cardiovascular system, balancing the pH of the skin, and preventing dehydration. Keeping the skin hydrated and balanced is one of the most important things you can do to ensure wedding glow. I recommend an infrared sauna because of the deep penetration and efficiency. Twenty minutes is all you need for desired results. Consult your doctor before using a sauna since in some cases it can exacerbate hypotension and cardiovascular issues.

On the opposite end of the spectrum, **CRYOTHERAPY** activates cold-shock proteins. This is a treatment that exposes your skin to subzero temperatures for a short period of time. It sounds excruciating, but it is actually refreshing. The time zips by quickly and you feel like a superhero afterward. The benefits include collagen production, cellulite reduction, and a quickened metabolism. This treatment can speed up the recovery of muscles during a new exercise routine. You can get similar benefits from a cold plunge, submerging your body into cold water for as long as 20 seconds; however, cryotherapy is much more comfortable. Consult your doctor before trying it.

MASSAGE THERAPY is exceptional for muscle tension, lymphatic flow, and overall circulation. There are many different massage styles, from deep tissue to light strokes. Massage has been proven to help ease anxiety and sleeplessness. A massage treatment can completely change your mindset and be very grounding. Find the style that works for you and go book an appointment. I recommend getting a massage the week before your wedding to reduce stress and ensure you're in a relaxed mindset leading up to the big day.

A **BACK TREATMENT** (sometimes referred to as a "back facial") is beneficial when experiencing acne on the shoulders and back. This treatment is carried out by an esthetician and involves all of the steps in a facial . . . on your back! Treatment is done while you are face down and helps to clear up any skin issues on the back while giving you an opportunity to learn how to better care for that area. It's the perfect choice if you plan to wear a wedding dress that exposes your arms and back.

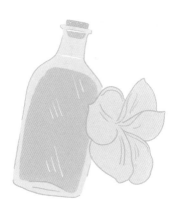

Common Ailments and At-Home Holistic Solutions

Skin conditions are common and do not always require professional treatments or prescriptions. Here are some remedies you can try at home.

As we've discussed, antioxidants protect against oxidative stress, which can cause melanin to be activated, which in turn can increase the likelihood of sun damage and **HYPERPIGMENTATION**. In addition to eating antioxidant-rich foods (think nuts, seeds, legumes, fruits, and vegetables), you can also use antioxidants on your face for additional benefits.

MELASMA is a hyperpigmentation that typically shows around the mouth, and sometimes on the forehead and cheeks. This is common during pregnancy and is often referred to as a "pregnancy mask," but in truth, anyone can experience this discoloration. When treating melasma, hormones typically need to be balanced internally. Visit your local naturopath or herbalist.

For **BLEMISHES**, honey is antibacterial and can cleanse as well as hydrate. Manuka honey, in particular, can work wonders when left on for 15 to 20 minutes. Avoid scrubbing at the skin to deter the spread of bacteria.

ECZEMA shows up as redness, flakiness, and sometimes spots, and is often itchy. It is diagnosed visually by

ANTIOXIDANT MASK

½ Tbsp raw,
organic honey

¼ tsp spirulina

¼ tsp crushed
chamomile

1. Mix the ingredients together and spread the mixture onto your skin.

2. Leave on for 10 to 15 minutes and remove with a warm towel.

a dermatologist. **PSORIASIS** is similar, but often involves scaling and a lot of flaking. I wish there was a true easy remedy for eczema or psoriasis. In most cases, there really is not, and the cause is often internal. Drink plenty of water, and eliminate fragrances and other triggers. Triggers can include diet, hormonal fluctuations, body temperature, and even physical contact with materials that irritate the skin. These ailments are not contagious. Use an herbal balm to soothe the affected areas.

ROSACEA is a benign disease, manifesting as redness, typically starting in the cheeks, and sometimes causing pustules and cysts. This disease is very common, affecting 5 percent of the population. It should also be treated internally, identifying and eliminating triggers. Staying cool and avoiding excessive heat or hot water when washing can help minimize redness.

CELLULITE affects almost everyone at some stage of their life. It looks like dimpling in the skin due to fat pushing through the loose connective tissue. A good coffee scrubbing can help smooth out skin. Coffee grounds help to break up fat deposits, and caffeine increases blood flow and constricts blood vessels, firming skin. Dry brushing can be used as a treatment or preventative measure. As

SPOT TREATMENT

½ tsp apple cider vinegar

½ tsp honey

¼ tsp cinnamon

¼ tsp cosmetic grade clay (found at your local health food store or online at mountainroseherbs .com)

1. Mix the ingredients together and apply the mixture directly onto the pimple.

2. Leave on for at least 20 minutes or overnight.

discussed on page 55, this practice creates detoxifying lymph movement. Try either of these methods, or a combination of both, every day for a week and note the results.

ROUGH, DRY SKIN can be easily remedied with an at-home scrub and/or dry brushing before showering. Do not scrub your skin if you have any open sores. Apply shea butter after towel drying for extra hydration. Shea butter is nourishing and locks in moisture (it should be used only on the body, not the face).

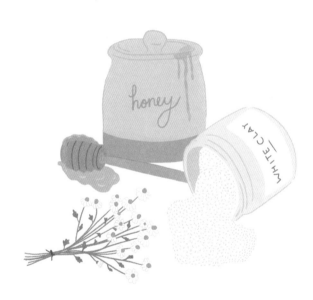

When to See a Dermatologist

Dermatologists are medical practitioners trained to diagnose and treat skin disorders. If you have moles, you should really be seeing a dermatologist once a year for a skin check to determine if any spots or moles look suspicious or cancerous. Separate from an annual skin check, it may be time to see a dermatologist if you have something that looks potentially dangerous (see ABCDEs of moles on page 112), or if you suffer from a persistent, ongoing skin issue and have exhausted all other treatment options. Dermatologists have an incredible depth of information and possess the knowledge to save lives.

However, some of these professionals can sometimes be a little prescription-happy. Prescription drugs, although very important in modern medicine, are oftentimes temporary solutions, meaning they soothe the symptoms of a condition, but unfortunately, do nothing to treat the root cause. For example, topical steroids are known to quickly obliterate skin irritations and reactions; however, the original symptoms can come back with a vengeance and even stronger than before, leading to new issues. Prescription acne treatments can clear skin but can also hinder your skin's ability to care for itself and stay nourished.

If you are in a pinch leading up to your wedding with a huge cystic pimple that will not go away, or an eczema breakout, and you have tried other remedies and nothing is working, this is the only time I would recommend seeing a dermatologist for a quick fix. In the long term, these cures do not address the root causes, which can sometimes be difficult or frustrating to figure out.

If you are looking for a dermatologist, get a recommendation from a friend or a trusted doctor. I do not recommend visiting a dermatologist casually; it is best to do your research, find one you like and can trust, and then stick with them. That way, they will get to know you and your skin over time and can make informed decisions based on your skin conditions.

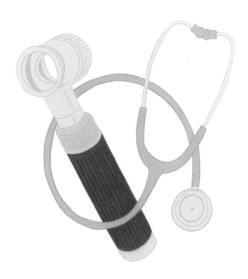

THE ABCDEs
OF MOLES

Here are the ABCDEs of moles—keep an eye out for these signs to help prevent the spread of skin cancer. While this outlines what to watch for, if any moles look alarming, please visit a dermatologist as soon as possible.

A = ASYMMETRY

Most melanomas are asymmetrical. Draw a line through the middle of a mole, and see if the two halves match. If they do, then it's likely a common mole. But if they don't, then you should get it checked out.

B = BORDER

Moles tend to have smooth, even borders. Melanomas often have uneven and scalloped or irregular borders.

C = COLOR

Various shades of brown, tan, or black in a single spot may be the first sign of melanoma. As melanomas progress, you may also see red, white, or blue in the spot. Comparatively, benign moles are usually one to two shades of brown.

D = DIAMETER OR DARK

The larger the spot, the greater the risk, since melanomas at the time of detection are usually about ¼ inch [6 mm] in diameter (although they can be smaller). Melanomas are often darker in color than benign moles. However, they can also be pink or colorless (amelanotic), although these kinds of melanomas are rare.

E = EVOLVING

Changes in size, shape, color, or height of a spot on your skin, as well as other changes, such as bleeding, itching, or crusting on a spot, may be warning signs of melanoma.

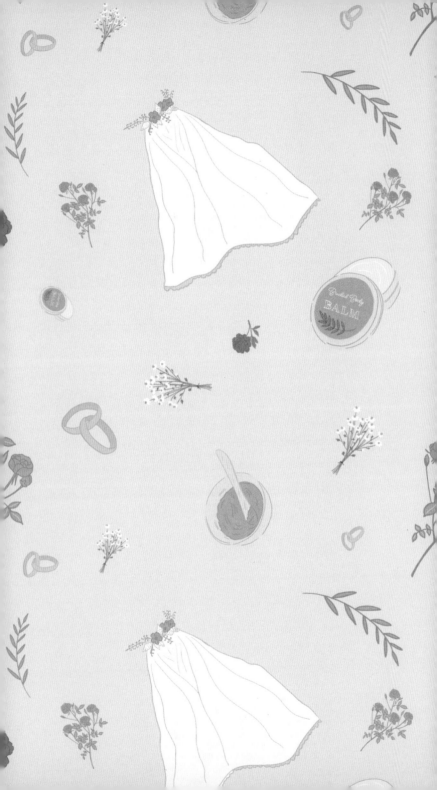

GETTING READY FOR THE WEDDING

Pre-ceremony preparation is an occasion to practice daily rituals that boost your skin's luminosity. During this time, keep in mind the skin health fundamentals: a regimen of supportive skin-care products, sufficient sleep, an exercise routine, and a well-balanced diet. If feasible, now is the perfect moment to indulge in some extra treatments to comfort both the body and mind. Do not forget that self-care can also happen in the moments in between—stop to pause and enjoy the little things.

Your wedding day, and the time leading up to it, is when everyone gets to show their love and appreciation for you, your partner, and your nuptials. It will be an amazing day. Here, I have included some ways to make pre-wedding skin care fun and to remedy hypothetical skin-care emergencies to ensure everything runs smoothly and you continue to glow on your big day.

Sharing the Glow

Skin care can be communal! Events like your bridal shower and bachelorette party can include glow-getting activities. Here are some ideas.

MAKE A DIY BODY SCRUB BAR. Set out ingredients and jars and allow guests to create their own scrub for their specific needs. Ingredients to include: oils (olive, coconut, almond, etc.), salt, sugar, honey, coffee grounds, oats, flower petals (rose, lavander, calendula). Use whatever makes you happiest!

VISIT A SPA. Some spas have communal pools, saunas, or other places to lounge, which are great places to socialize between massages or other treatments.

GROUP GUA SHA. Ask your local gua sha expert to host a party so you can learn a fun, new skin-care routine alongside your bridal party. If this is not something your local gua sha technician does, buy the tools and host your own!

TREATMENTS WITH FRIENDS. In lieu of bridal shower gifts, ask friends and family to join you for one of the treatments listed in the Professional Treatments section on page 87. Even better—maybe they'll offer to pay for you! If you make a day of it, this can be a fun way to spend some quality time together and help supplement the cost of treatments.

The Month Before

Your wedding is a month away. Are you excited?! Here are a few things to keep in mind in the run-up to the big day.

ESTABLISH AND FOLLOW YOUR ROUTINES. Since the big day is right around the corner, hopefully you have all your skin-care routines established by now, but if not, it's not too late to start. This is the time to enforce—and stick to—your morning and nightly routines. Don't skip them!

DO NOT INTRODUCE NEW PRODUCTS. If you can avoid it, do not change your skin-care products at this time; it is best to keep using whatever it is you have been using. Heightened excitement means heightened levels of cortisol and a higher likelihood of a skin reaction, so avoiding new ingredients is best. Feel free to increase your masking, and perhaps treat yourself to some extra exfoliation.

SUN PROTECTION. Pre-wedding gatherings are often hosted outdoors. Try to avoid overexposure to the sun these few weeks, but if you are outside for an extended period, do your best to remember sun protection. Consider stashing a mineral sunscreen in your purse for easy access when you're out and about.

DE-STRESS. You will probably be tying up plenty of loose ends and making last-minute arrangements and final decisions. Plan the time necessary for self-care and take it easy. Exercise, meditate, etc. (refer to page 81 for more ideas on stress management). Your wedding is an important day, but maintain perspective. Keep in touch with yourself and your immediate needs and enjoy the process.

The Week Before

DRINK WATER! It takes 3 days to get fully hydrated, so now is the time! Drink half your weight in ounces (or kilograms) daily and use electrolytes when needed.

DO NOT SACRIFICE YOUR EXERCISE. Keeping a routine will ensure your sanity during this time.

EXFOLIATE! Slough off dead surface skin cells and even out skin tone with either a manual or chemical exfoliant.

PARTAKE IN SOME AT-HOME FACIAL MASSAGE with either your hands, a gua sha tool, or a jade roller. This will create blood flow, stimulate elastin, and boost collagen.

Make sure you are getting plenty of time to **REST AND RELAX**, whether it be through massage or sleep.

MASK IT UP! You should mask 2 or 3 times this week.

Now would be a great time to get a **BODY TREATMENT**, like a scrub, mud bath, or wrap.

Hopefully, your **FINAL FACIAL** can be scheduled during this week, with the guidance of your esthetician.

The Night Before

DON'T DRINK TOO MUCH ALCOHOL. It can be tempting to (over)indulge if you're having a rehearsal dinner or welcome party where alcohol is offered and everyone is in a celebratory mood. Enjoy yourself, but remember that tomorrow is the big day, and you want to look and feel your best! (If you had a little too much, turn to page 121 for a morning-after recovery routine.)

SCRUB with a body scrub of your choosing and moisturize with a balm or oil.

EXFOLIATE and apply a hydration mask before bed.

Get plenty of **BEAUTY SLEEP!**

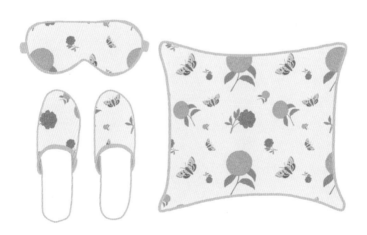

On the Big Day

It's finally here! Now is the time to celebrate your nuptials and enjoy this event with your closest friends and family.

Here are some tips to keep you glowing on your wedding day.

- Exercise away any pre-wedding jitters.

- Post workout, shower and follow your normal skin-care routine.

- If you're getting your makeup done, show up with a clean face and let them work their magic. Wash your skin and tone, moisturize, etc., like you normally do, but do not apply any makeup.

- If you are doing your own makeup, consider using a light mica product. Mica powders are made from ground-up mineral mica, and therefore appear sparkly, like very fine glitter. Mica can be used to create an all-over glow and sparkle, or to highlight areas such as your cheekbones, collarbones, and shoulders.

- If you are going makeup free, wear that glow loud and proud.

- Breathe deeply, stay hydrated, and enjoy yourself!

Did you drink too much at your rehearsal dinner? It's easy to do when you're having a blast and surrounded by people you love! Don't fret!

Here is a tried-and-true recovery routine.

1. Cleanse your face using your usual cleanser and cold water.

2. Apply a hyaluronic acid–based hydrating or honey mask.

3. After the mask, actively massage your daily eye product (refer to the eye massage on page 36) into your skin, creating blood flow and "waking" up your skin.

4. Gua sha, jade roll, or massage your face from jawbone to collarbone in a light, sweeping motion. These movements will activate the lymphatic system and you'll instantly de-puff.

5. Cool cucumber slices or an eye mask can soothe puffiness and firm your skin.

6. Finally, hydrate with electrolytes, and supplement with B vitamins.

Dealing with Skin Emergencies

Skin emergencies happen. They are rare and might simply be a part of your wedding story. Don't panic. It may feel like a disaster, but chances are no one will notice and you will not remember 5 years from now. Luckily, there are solutions to help lessen the effects so you can focus on enjoying your big day.

SUNBURN

So you got too much sun and ended up with a sunburn — ouch! Too much UV sunlight can penetrate and burn your skin; this process can take less than 10 minutes. If you get a sunburn, a cool to lukewarm bath with finely ground oats and chamomile will help soothe the fire (see recipe on facing page). Layer on cool compresses and aloe; avoid popping any blisters or scrubbing any peeling skin. On your body, moisturize with a heavy oil, like apricot or coconut oil. On your face, use an increased amount of your facial moisturizer. Drink extra water to keep cells functioning and speed up repair.

PIMPLE

If you get a pimple, **DO NOT POP IT!** Use ice to cool the inflammation and take down any swelling. Use a spot treatment to exfoliate and calm your skin. A concealer or your makeup artist will be your best friend today. Refer to page 23 for additional tips.

For either of these hiccups, a mineral makeup will help combat the rough texture. Color correcting will help neutralize the discoloration and redness. You can use a green concealer to counter redness, and a purple one to counter yellow undertones. My personal wedding makeup artist and good friend, Kirsten Coleman, suggests, "Always test bridal makeup with photos—both with a flash and without." If you have a professional photographer, they may even be able to edit your blemish away.

SOOTHING BATH

1 cup [100 g] dry rolled oats

¼ cup [10 g] dried chamomile (a couple tea bags work!)

1. Add the ingredients to a bathtub full of cool to lukewarm water.

2. Soak for 15 minutes.

3. After bathing and patting skin dry, immediately apply an occlusive body moisturizer, like shea butter or apricot oil. This locks in moisture and ensures hydration.

HAVE THE
BEST DAY EVER!

Weddings are a time when everyone wants to look their best. And you absolutely will. Maintain gratitude for what you love about your skin, yourself, your partner, and all of the beautiful people coming together to celebrate your commitments to a lifetime of love.

Settling on a skin-care regimen, establishing some form of regular body movement, and managing dietary triggers can all be challenges to getting started, but doing any and all of these practices daily will lead to great rewards. Skin care is self-care and self-care is self-love. Remember to be patient with and attentive to your skin—it is a living thing, just like a plant. If you water and care for it, it will grow and thrive and show you what healthy looks like. Glow is whole body—it comes from feeling so vibrant that you radiate wellness.

The skin is a fascinating, complex instrument. When your skin is not looking the way you would like, remember that our skin cells turn over and are replaced every moon cycle. We are connected to the earth and are constantly given new chances to start fresh and undo the damage done along the way. The skin is an organ with the capability to renew itself. It does so in conjunction with other body systems, and our daily habits can advance or hinder that restoration. Even when you think you are not glowing, **YOU ARE GLOWING**. Your skin is working for you constantly, helping you feel the world around you, maintaining your body temperature, and protecting you from harm. Love it all, freckles, moles, blemishes, and scars—it's all a part of you. Embrace it as you celebrate finding love in this wild world.

I hope by now you are glowing a bit more and feeling ready for your wedding! No matter the state your skin is in, do not forget that glow is more than skin deep; it comes from an inner vitality projecting itself out and into the world. When you feel good, it shows.

RESOURCES

FAVORITE BRANDS

SKIN CARE

Biophilia Botanicals
biophiliabotanicals.com

Botnia
botniaskincare.com

Chuck & Sam
chuckandsam.com

Heart of Gold
heartofgold.love

Honua Hawaiian Skincare
honuaskincare.com

Laurel
laurelskin.com

Wild Hill Botanicals
wildhillbotanicals.com

MAKEUP

Kjaer Weis
kjaerweis.com

RMS Beauty
rmsbeauty.com

Vapour
vapourbeauty.com

W3ll People
w3llpeople.com

BOOKS

An Atlas of Natural Beauty: Botanical Ingredients for Retaining and Enhancing Beauty by Victoire de Taillac and Ramdane Touhami

Herbs for Natural Beauty: Create Your Own Herbal Shampoos, Cleansers, Creams, Bath Blends, and More by Rosemary Gladstar

Medical Herbalism: The Science and Practice of Herbal Medicine by David Hoffman

Power of the Seed: Your Guide to Oils for Health & Beauty by Susan M. Parker

Younger Skin Starts in the Gut: 4-Week Program to Identify and Eliminate Your Skin-Aging Triggers by Nigma Talib

WEBSITES

Beauty Heroes
beauty-heroes.com
Shop clean beauty.

BLK + GRN
blkgrn.com
Buy green wellness products and support black women–owned businesses.

Mountain Rose Herbs
mountainroseherbs.com
A great source for sustainable herbs and oils. (However, I always recommend trying your local health food store or herb shop first!)

Skin Cancer Foundation
skincancer.org
Information on the prevention, early detection, and treatment of skin cancer.

ACKNOWLEDGMENTS

I have so much gratitude to everyone who helped this idea come to fruition. This was an endeavor for me and I could not have done it without a support system (in no order, because all of you are amazing).

Huge thank-you to the team at Chronicle Books for all of the guidance. Specifically to editor Deanne Katz for inviting me into the writing world and encouraging me on this journey. Special thank-you to Claire Gilhuly and everyone else for your much-needed feedback. Seeta Roy, I am so grateful for your beautiful illustrations. And thank you to Rachel Hiles for thinking of me.

Thank you to my family, Mom, Dad, Cyn, Terri, Jerry, and the rest of our growing clan B+E+C, C+J, RJ+J. I appreciate your patience, love, and support.

Knowledge is nothing if not shared, and I would like to acknowledge the teachers in this industry who compassionately imparted their wisdom: Kim Riley Rowser, Alice Duvernell, Christy Swenson, Monique McDonald, Lindsay Flint, Cecily Braden, Kristin Shaw, Laurel Shaffer, Angela Peck, Mitcho Thompson, all the teachers at California School of Herbal Studies, Gay Lee Gulbrandson, and Anne Branham. I would also like to acknowledge all of the ancient teachers and cultures who have generously shared their remedies, techniques, and theories.

I have been inspired by my teachers, and also have been lucky to have personal expanders who have shown me what manifestation is. Thank you Elizabeth Markham, Katie Woods, Kirsten Coleman, Justine Kahn, Tara Salem, and Donni Davy. I am in constant awe and value each of you so much. Thank you for your help.

To my clients, Reboot Float Spa, Ride Oakland, and Timeless Coffee, you guys rock!

And so many thank-yous to my partner, Scott. I could not have done any of this without your warm meals, endless encouragement, brushing Barney's teeth, and forever picking up after me. Being your bride is the best.